A BLUEPRINT FOR RADIANT HEALTH AND WELLNESS

REVOLUTIONIZING YOUR HEALTH

*Getting Beyond the Programming
of Big Medicine*

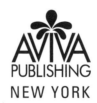

AVIVA
PUBLISHING
NEW YORK

Marvin Kunikiyo, D.C.

Revolutionizing Your Health

Getting Beyond the Programming of Big Medicine

©2010 by Marvin Kunikiyo, D.C.

Address all inquiries to:

Dr. Marvin Kunikiyo

P.O.Box 3082

Yelm, WA 98597

(360) 292-3711

www.RevolutionizingYourHealth.com

ISBN: 978-1-935586-06-7

Library of Congress Control Number: 2010902174

Editor: Tyler R. Tichelaar, Ph.D.

Cover Photo: Clark Little Photography

Cover Design & Interior Layout: Fusion Creative Works, www.fusioncw.com

Printed in the United States of America

For additional copies, visit: www.RevolutionizingYourHealth.com

DISCLAIMER

Although this book is based on true events, all names, places, and events have been fictionalized, modified or changed completely to protect the innocent and the guilty, without implying either. Characters, institutions, corporations, and organizations are either products of the imagination or, if real, used fictitiously without any intent to describe their actual conduct, thoughts, physical characteristics, intentions, backgrounds, or medical conditions. Any similarity to actual people, events, or location is not intentional. This book is solely intended for educational purposes. Any medical description or what may appear to be medical advice is not meant to be represented as accurate, safe, or, in some cases, even remotely possible. If you need medical or psychological care, please seek the help of a competent health care practitioner. It is never safe to self-diagnose. Any recommendations are the personal opinion of the author.

CONTENTS

FOREWORD

In a world of advanced medical technology, do you wonder, like me, why the health of Americans is declining? Do you know how to navigate the sea of information to learn what you need to do to stay healthy? How does the notion that the medicine to "cure" could also harm you in a myriad of ways sit with you? I find it disturbing. I find it disturbing that in my practice of eye healthcare, I have patients asking me to give them the "medicine" that made their friends' eyes so much better. "You know, the one that is advertised on TV." It was somewhat of an oddity to me when drugs began to be advertised on television because I remember when it was no longer acceptable to advertise alcohol on TV because "young people would be exposed to it."

We have become a culture in which we must have, and in fact, we demand a pill to make us feel better. We expect a quick fix, and we expect our doctors to have all the answers. The problem is that doctors don't have all the answers, and I know this because I am one of them. I have also been a patient, and I know what it is like to hurt and desperately to want something, anything, to make the pain go away.

It has been relatively recently that society has accepted more alternative forms of medicine (chiropractic, massage, biofeedback, acupuncture, etc.) as mainstream. It is also important to note that as recently as the 1920s, archaic medical practices were still accepted and being performed. As the science of medicine grew and developed over the years, what was new and innovative was often regarded as unacceptable. It is easy to see as we look back at history that it is difficult to get a group of people to break free from the mode of thinking in which they have been indoctrinated, even if it is no longer their best option. Going against the popular choices can feel a lot like swimming upstream. As a collective, we are not so willing to change because of fear of the unknown.

Most people tend to make health choices and decisions based on propaganda and word-of-mouth recommendations derived from hearsay more than facts. When it comes to your health, why would you take someone else's word for it as opposed to doing your own homework and making the best-educated decision that is right for you? Someone may go bungee jumping and think it's the most fantastic, exhilarating experience of his life and tell you that you absolutely must try it. You reason, "Well, it looks pretty scary, but if it's fantastic and exhilarating I'd like that, too, so what the heck?" Unfortunately, when your jump leads to a broken arm, your experience is the polar opposite of your friend's. While this example may seem extreme, consider for a moment how an innocuous-sounding pretty pink pill in the ad with the flowers blooming, the sun shining, and the smiling, happy people could be a bad thing? For starters, how about the list of potential side effects that reads like the credits that roll on and on at the end of a movie? We become hypnotized by what we want to hear to the point that we tune out what we don't want to hear. You might argue that the pretty pink pill is a way out of your illness, pain, and disease. After all, experts are giving us this information, and surely they only have your best interests at heart. But do they?

It is time to change the way we look at our health and take a more personal, dynamic, and vocal role in it. If we are to revolutionize the way we think about our health and our health and wellness care, the first step is to gain the knowledge that will allow us to be informed consumers and make the best choices for ourselves. That is where this book comes in.

In this book you will find, in a very readable, accessible format, a treasure trove of information, some of which may come as such a surprise that it will change the way you look at health and healthcare. The author, Dr. Marvin Kunikiyo, is a knowledgeable, compassionate and revolutionary healthcare professional. He has drawn upon his twenty-four years of experience in patient care, his personal experiences, and the research and knowledge he has gained over the years to provide you with the information and the tools that will, literally, revolutionize your health. He takes us through causes of disease (like high blood pressure and heart disease), asthma, what the big deal about salt is (or is not), the importance of water in ways you have probably never heard, the dark and light sides of nutrition, the vaccine controversy, and so much more. He also describes what you can do if you are someone who suffers from an affliction or illness or are someone who simply wants to maintain wonderful health.

We are at a point in our world's evolution where it is no longer acceptable to sit back and let everyone else make decisions for us. As Dr. Kunikiyo says, with knowledge, there is power. This book provides you with the basis to start asking more questions and to make choices that serve you, involve you, and are the best for you, rather than your just accepting someone else's dictum.

Certainly, if you were working on your car and something fell into your eye, you would want a trained professional to remove it for you. If you were in an accident, you would want the technology and skills of a trauma center and a trained emergency physician. This book fills in the gaps between the extremes of emergency care and health maintenance and wellness. Everyone should have the knowledge contained in this book.

The term "holistic medicine" is thrown around quite casually these days, but what does it really mean? The typical definition implies treating the person as a "whole" with emphasis on the connection between the body and the mind. Holistic medicine has more to do with wellness and engaging those wellness practices that maintain a person's health integrity and less to do with fitting a list of symptoms into a program that can give a name to your problem and spit out a standard, medically acceptable, treatment plan. Today, medicine claims to be more holistic—and some really wonderful, truly holistic healthcare facilities, physicians, and establishments are out there— but that still remains the exception rather than the norm. In many respects, it's still an uphill battle, but why should it be? Isn't it the goal of healthcare providers to assist a fellow human to be as healthy and well as he or she possibly can be?

Dr. Kunikiyo's book takes us beyond convention and generally held beliefs. It is a welcome breath of fresh air from the oppression of what we have been led to believe is the truth about health and wellness care. It is, indeed, time for a revolution. What you don't know can hurt you and the ones you love. It's time for a change.

Laurie Pyne

Dr. Laurie Pyne

INTRODUCTION

Knowledge is power.

Currently a big debate is being waged over healthcare reform. The media and politicians are stirring the pot, whipping the public into a frenzy over this issue. Lobbyists for the pharmaceutical companies, the AMA, and the insurance industry are hard at work, jockeying for position. The call for all Americans to have health insurance coverage righteously drones on.

But is this reform *really* the solution to our healthcare system's woes? We already spend more money per capita than any other nation in the world, and yet the United States is one of the world's sickest nations. If we're already spending more on healthcare than any other nation, and we are nowhere near the top in terms of health, I suggest we need more than just healthcare reform. We need a health revolution!

What about you? Are you satisfied with your level of health? Do you have enough energy to do the things you want to do? Are your daily activities restricted by pain and illness, so that you're unable to do the things you really enjoy doing? Perhaps you're even unable to work due to pain or illness. Has the joy gone out of your life because your body is unhappy with you, and it is letting you know it? Are you currently taking several medications on an ongoing basis? Have you been told that if you don't take this or that pill (usually for high blood pressure or cholesterol) you're going to die? So you take the pills, but you still feel lousy (probably even lousier)! What kind of healthcare is that?

So what do I mean by saying we need more than just healthcare reform? Healthcare reform simply means a re-distribution of money at the top. At best, it will provide sub-par healthcare to more people. Sub-par, as you know, is only a good thing if you're playing golf.

A health revolution, on the other hand, means changing the approach to treating illness and promoting good health. Consider the days of bloodletting and frontal lobotomies. Looking back now, those seem like ludicrous procedures. But at the time, they were well accepted as being beneficial to the patient. Fortunately, new knowledge comes, and what seemed to be "cutting edge" (pun intended) is now viewed as obsolete and primitive.

But what if a society gets stuck on an outdated, obsolete, ineffective approach to health and healthcare? What if the people who are putting out the propaganda (beliefs surrounding health and healthcare) really care about the money more than they care about your health? Just as an example, before 1920, coronary heart disease was so rare in the United States that when Dr. Paul Dudley White, at the time a young intern, introduced the German electrocardiograph to his fellow doctors at Harvard University, they told him he should instead focus on a branch of medicine that would be more profitable. [1] Imagine how poor our care of heart disease would be today if Dr. White had listened to them—fortunately, Dr. White cared about his patients' health over putting money in his own pocket!

Today, the pharmaceutical companies have a lot to gain by keeping the public ignorant, and a lot to lose if people wake up to the truth. The truth is that drugs are making people sicker and killing people more than helping them. The world of healthcare has become *iatrogenic*, a word that means illness or death caused by medical intervention. In a *Washington Post* article from April 15, 1998, Rick Weiss reported:

> More than 2 million Americans become seriously ill every year because of toxic reactions to *correctly prescribed* medicines *taken properly*, and 106,000 die from those reactions, a new study concludes. That surprisingly high number makes drug side effects at least the sixth, and perhaps even the fourth, most common cause of death in this country.

Could it be true that drugs are causing more harm than good? Would we be healthier as a nation if we looked to the cause of disease, rather than trying to suppress symptoms of illness?

Our current healthcare paradigm is severely flawed because it is based on a faulty premise. The medical paradigm sees the body as an unintelligent mass, and it holds that we have to make it do what we think it should be doing through the action of pharmaceutical drugs. This belief is the root of the problem. My question is, "When did we become smarter than the Intelligence that made the body?"

True healthcare looks to the cause of disease, and it makes the proper corrections. Most (physical) causes of disease are due either to a nutrient deficiency or a harmful agent taken into the body, or both.

If your car had a water deficiency, would you give it chemicals (drugs) to prevent it from overheating? Of course not; you'd give it water! Your body is no different. If it's low on water and you give it drugs instead to suppress any symptoms of dehydration, your body will develop inflammation. Inflammation, or *inflammare* in Latin, literally means "to set on fire." Sounds a lot like what your car looks like when it (is water deficient and) overheats.

There's a reason why your body develops certain symptoms. It's the body's response to dealing with a problem, usually a nutrient deficiency or a harmful substance in the body. Does modern medicine take this into account at all? No. Because if it did, a LOT less prescription drug consumption would take place, and that would be disastrous not only to the pharmaceutical companies, but ultimately to the medical profession as well.

My initial idea and inspiration for writing this book came as a result of my suffering seasonal allergies for about ten years, only to have the ailment completely resolved after drinking ionized water for about a month. I also noticed that canker sores that had plagued me for the last year or two (and were increasing in frequency and intensity) also disappeared. My digestion and elimination improved significantly. My energy level shot up. Additionally, I was filled with a feeling of well-being that I hadn't experienced in a long time. How did this happen? I had to know. This started my research into ionized water and its effects on health.

As I researched, I came across other books and articles that all seemed to point in a similar direction, and simultaneously, my book began to expand and become more focused until it has now become a comprehensive book on health. It has been my intention that this book will be very concise, easy to understand, and will hold the reader's interest. A lengthy book filled with too many medical terms can be intimidating, difficult to comprehend, and sometimes even boring. This book is, therefore, purposely on the shorter side, yet quite thorough, and it should give the reader ample knowledge and understanding to make a total revolution in his or her health.

I want to acknowledge all of the researchers, scientists, physicians and authors mentioned and/or quoted in this book. Many of them have done extensive research into their specific fields of interest, and this book has been built on their efforts. I have simply sorted out and rearranged the information in my own head to present it to you, the reader, in a clear way that hopefully captures your attention. Many of the books and articles resourced here are recommended to those who want to learn more on specific topics.

Throughout the book, I will frequently refer to the programming we have received from Big Medicine, and I will give specific examples of that programming. So much misinformation has been programmed into us that we don't even realize we may be operating from a foundation of false information. In building a house, the foundation has to be precise. Even a half-inch off the mark at the bottom may result in walls that are way off at the top. Similarly, if you start with a foundation of faulty information and false beliefs surrounding health, then radiant health and wellness will forever elude you (just like straight walls).

The only way a health revolution can occur is for people to wake up from Big Medicine's brainwashing and start taking responsibility for their own health. Instead of medicating every single symptom, we need knowledge to determine which nutrient deficiency or harmful substance is causing distress to the body, so we can make the proper correction.

My approach and intention in writing this book is to provide readers with enough knowledge in the form of statistics, physiology, and often pure reason to get them to think and start to question the status quo. There's just one problem. Most people are pretty lazy—too lazy to think on their own. They rely on what others (mainly the media and medical doctors) tell them. And understandably, it is a tremendous amount of work to understand how the body functions, and to learn how to care for it properly, which is precisely why I wrote this book to give readers the information they need in a compacted form. Another hurdle to self-responsibility for one's health is fear. "If I don't take this medication, the doctor says I'm likely to die of a heart attack." "If I don't vaccinate my children, they may die of swine flu (every year it's a different flu virus, isn't it?); I'd feel like I wasn't a responsible parent, and I might be responsible for my children's death." The programming runs deep. I attempt to paint the clearest picture possible so you can see beyond the "Kool Aid" programming of Big Medicine. And believe me, most of us have drunk the Kool Aid.

Taking back responsibility for your health requires knowledge—of how your body works, what causes disease, and what leads to radiant health. The only way a person will be able to transcend the dogma and fear instilled by Big Medicine is absolutely to know the causes of disease. When you absolutely know that cholesterol is not the cause of heart disease, why would you even consider taking Lipitor? When you absolutely know that vaccines not only do not prevent disease, but actually cause disease, choosing not to vaccinate your child becomes the obvious wise choice. This book provides the knowledge you need to do just that—get beyond the programming of Big Medicine.

You *can* understand how your body works. You *can* understand what causes disease and what gives rise to health. It doesn't take being a genius or a rocket scientist to understand this information. So please, as you get set to read this book, allow yourself to know and understand.

It is my sincere hope that this book will **empower** you with enough knowledge that you will take back responsibility for and control of your own health. After all, you deserve to experience **radiant health and wellness**.

Marvin Kunikiyo

Marvin Kunikiyo, D.C.

PART ONE

GETTING BEYOND THE
PROGRAMMING OF BIG MEDICINE

This book is divided into two sections. Part One is designed to move the reader beyond the programming of Big Medicine by clearly demonstrating its flawed approach. Once you are equipped with enough knowledge to give up your reliance on Big Medicine, you are ready to be filled with knowledge to empower you toward self-responsibility.

One of my patients had an experience that perfectly illustrates the value of self-responsibility. He was cutting branches off a tree when some of the tree's very poisonous sap got in his eye. This man owns a water ionizer machine, so he went into his house to try to flush it out with ionized water. (If you don't know about ionized water, don't worry—you will by the end of this book—it may be the most important thing you learn here). The ionized water didn't seem to reduce his pain at all, so his wife quickly went on the Internet and searched for information about the tree and its sap. She discovered that the sap normally causes blindness when it gets in the eye because of its very acidic make-up. She immediately set their water ionizer to the highest alkaline setting and then doused his eye with the more alkaline water. Instant relief! The pain and inflammation quickly subsided, and to this day, he can still see perfectly.

This patient later found out that virtually all other such cases resulted in blindness, even with immediate medical attention. (MDs apparently don't know that a strong base—an alkaline—can neutralize a strong acid.) Even if they did figure that out, no hospital I know of in the U.S. has a water ionizer. With all of the fancy, expensive, high-tech gadgets hospitals have, they choose not to have water ionizers. By comparison, 80% of Japanese hospitals do have water ionizers. Most people in this man's position would have had their wives drive them to the emergency room or have immediately called 911, and then have waited in agony until the ambulance came. Once he was at the hospital, the man would have been subjected to a medical doctor routinely trying to flush out his eye with a saline solution (typically neutral in pH), which would have done absolutely nothing for him, and he would have ended up blind in one eye.

This man and his wife had enough knowledge to figure out that the best thing for him was to neutralize the acidic sap with a strong alkaline fluid. Most importantly, he chose to think for himself. That's why he can still see perfectly out of that eye when virtually everyone else exposed to that sap would lose his vision.

My desire is for you to become like this man—empowered with knowledge and unafraid to think for yourself. A big gap exists between really understanding something and just collecting information. If you are in the habit of simply collecting information, it will probably not do you any good because you're not applying that information to your life. When you truly understand something, the natural extension of that knowledge is to apply it to your life, just as this man did.

Consider this book to be an owner's manual for your body. Strive to understand every concept in it, and don't be afraid to go back and reread or consult it as needed. It will not make your head spin with medical terminology, but instead, it is written for the layperson to understand. If there's something you don't completely grasp, read it again. In the end, you'll be very happy you did.

CHAPTER ONE

HEALTHCARE VS. SICKNESS CARE

*I firmly believe that if the entire materia medica
(prescription drugs) as now used could be sunk to the bottom of the
sea, it would be all the better for mankind—
and all the worse for the fishes.*
— **Oliver Wendell Holmes**

In this first chapter, you will become aware of some fairly incriminating evidence against Big Medicine. My intention is not to degrade or discredit anyone, but rather to compel the reader to decide to become self-responsible. If the current people and the Big Medicine system you rely upon for your healthcare and your health (they're not always the same thing) are failing you, and they clearly do not have your best interest at heart, why would you want to continue to rely on that system? Why not choose to become empowered with knowledge, and fearlessly make your own health choices? I hope this chapter truly wakes you up to the reality of healthcare in this country.

The U.S. is the world's wealthiest nation, it spends the most on healthcare, and yet it is ranked #37 in healthcare in the world. Current estimates put spending on healthcare in the United States at approximately 16% of gross domestic product. In 2007, an estimated $2.26 trillion was spent on healthcare in the United States, or $7,439 per person. A recent study found that medical expenditure was the cause for 60% of all personal bankruptcies in the United States.

The United States and Canada account for 48% of world pharmaceutical sales, while Europe, Japan, and all other nations account for 30%, 9%, and 13%, respectively. [1]

We're spending more money on pharmaceutical drugs than the rest of the world, and yet we're sicker. That should be a big clue!

When are we going to wake up as a nation and realize that drugs are making us sicker?

Japan, meanwhile, is ranked #1 in the world for health and longevity. What do the Japanese know that we don't? Many possible factors are responsible for this difference. One likely reason may be that the Japanese consume a diet with more whole foods and less processed foods. Another lesser known fact is that in Japan, 1 in 5 households have a water ionizer in their homes. Most Americans have never heard of ionized water. In Japan, a water ionizer called Kangen Water™ has been approved for use as a medical device in hospitals by the Japanese Ministry of Health. Most hospitals (80%) in Japan now have and use these machines to help treat many diseases. One of the first things hospitals do is to check the patient's pH. Your pH is the level of your body's acidity or alkalinity; it is measured on a scale where 7 represents neutrality and anything lower than that is increasingly acidic while higher numbers measure alkalinity. These changes of acidity and alkalinity are based on the hydrogen-ion concentration or hydrogen-ion activity of your body, or of a solution, such as water, or the tree sap I mentioned in the story earlier. Ideally, our bodies should have a pH of roughly 7.0 to 7.4, with slight variance depending on the individual. A water ionizer helps to neutralize acids and alkalizes the body to maintain a healthy pH balance. Because many diseases have their root in an acidic body, ionized, alkaline water is given to bring the patient's pH to a more optimal level. Drugs are used only as a last resort.

In the U.S., drugs are usually the first (and often the only) treatment option. We simply medicate people to death. One drug creates a host of side effects, which then requires other drugs to combat those side effects, and on and on. Not to mention the toxic effects on the liver and kidneys. Look at any drug ad in a magazine—the list of side effects, complications, and precautions make up most of the text in the advertisement. Often, one of the possible side effects is the very thing the drug was supposed to prevent!

Eleanor McBean, N.D., provides in her excellent book *The Poisoned Needle,* some statistics that give a different view of our sad state of health and healthcare:

INCREASE IN KILLER DISEASES DURING THE PAST 70 YEARS....

- Insanity increased 400%

- Cancer increased 308%

- Anemia increased 300%

- Epilepsy increased 397%

- Bright's Disease increased 65%

- Heart Disease increased 179%

- Diabetes increased 1800% (In spite of or because of insulin)

- Polio increased 680%

Dr. McBean concludes from this information, "Never in the history of this country have preventable diseases flourished with such wild abandon, continuously being fed by the very drugs and commercialized irritants that set them into operation in the first place." [2]

Clearly, something needs to change. But what is it? Why is our "health" care system failing us?

I want to make a distinction between healthcare and sickness care. Our medical system is not truly healthcare. To me, health "care" means to enhance and improve one's health either by learning your body's requirements for optimal health and giving your body what it needs, or by finding the cause of disease and correcting the problem. An excellent example of this process is chiropractic care. Chiropractors find the cause of the problem—spinal joint dysfunction that causes nerve interference—and they correct the spinal joint dysfunction through a specific adjustment, thereby removing the nerve interference or nerve pressure. By contrast, the medical approach first would be drugs to suppress the symptoms. This treatment often includes steroid injections, which are known to cause joint destruction. During the years I've been in practice, I've heard of so many joints that have been rendered useless through the use of repeated steroid injections. Next, commonly known as pre-surgery, physical therapy is attempted. Then if that fails, surgery is often recommended to cut out the offending structure, often a herniated disc or calcium deposits (the effect of long standing spinal joint dysfunction).

In a society addicted to feeling good now and "quick fixes," drugs are a great solution, seemingly. But all drugs usually do is suppress the symptoms. The symptoms are there for a reason. They are the body's way of saying, "Help! Do something!"

I remember once watching "The Oprah Winfrey Show" when the topic was traumatic life-threatening injuries. The person who caught my interest was an attorney, who had been shot multiple times in the throat and chest at close range on the courthouse steps by a gunman with a grudge. The attorney managed to get behind a tree and dodge most of the bullets until the man's gun was empty and he could be tackled. The attorney, upon reflecting on the incident, marveled that he had felt no pain during the incident until half an hour later when the ambulance was taking him to the hospital.

Oprah asked the guest medical doctor why the attorney wouldn't feel any pain right away. The doctor replied that it was because the attorney already knew the cause of his injury, so he needed to mobilize all of his energy into surviving. His body pumped itself full of endorphins so he could survive the assault by playing "dodge bullet." The medical doctor added that if the lawyer had been shot in the back, he probably would have felt pain immediately because his body wouldn't know what had hit him. I loved the doctor's next statement: "Pain is our body's alarm system, alerting us to a problem we need to address."

So many people look at pain as an annoyance, rather than the body's cry for help. The medical approach is to suppress "annoying symptoms," rather than trying to find the cause of them. Even medicine's attempts at "preventive care" are misguided, as you'll see later when I discuss heart disease. Sickness care treats the symptoms (usually by suppressing them), but true healthcare looks to the cause of the distressing symptoms, and then it attempts to correct the cause.

The point I want to make here is that our current approach to health isn't working very well. It's a crisis care approach (which is why I call it sickness care). It totally **ignores** the **cause** of the patient's ill health, and overmedicates people, making them sicker and sicker.

Let me tell you a little about my own journey in health and sickness. To say I was not the healthiest child would be a bit of an understatement. In addition to asthma and allergies, I was also "sick" a lot with the common cold or flu. In my teenage years, I can remember getting sick almost every other month, with my cold symptoms lasting usually one to two weeks. I would go to the medical doctor, get my antibiotics—which by the way means "against life"—take them religiously, and still be sick for usually two weeks. After a while, I began to wonder what good (if any) the antibiotics were really doing me. So the next time I got sick, I purposely neglected going to the doctor. Same result. The cold still lasted one to two weeks before it resolved on its own. However, I soon began to notice that my "colds" were getting farther and farther apart as I continued to stay away from the medical doctor and antibiotics. By the time I graduated from high school, my colds were down to once or twice a year. At present, I can't remember the last time I had a cold—it's been years. When I come into contact with sick (infectious) patients or other people, I don't have the least concern of "catching" their infections because I now know that an infection is just one of the body's ways of cleaning house. I also know that sickness only occurs when the body is burdened with excess toxins and acidity, or when the immune system is worn down from mental or emotional stress. In other words, bacteria and viruses only thrive in an unclean environment. As within, so without—and vice versa; just as smallpox could only thrive in unsanitary conditions, and it declined as sanitary conditions improved, a clean internal environment has no place for the establishment of disease (infection) and no need for house cleaning (the outward symptoms of infection). Furthermore, I know from experience that antibiotics only serve to weaken the immune system; I have not taken a single antibiotic since high school, and my immune system has obviously gotten stronger.

Let's now turn our attention to the "gatekeepers" for your healthcare. "Health" insurance companies don't care about your health. They are a "for-profit" business, a middleman who wants his piece of the pie. What service are these companies actually providing for that piece of the pie (besides "regulating" your healthcare)? It's like the commercial where the man takes control at the scene of an accident and someone says, "Boy I'm so glad you happened to be here, Doc!" The man replies, "Oh, I'm not a doctor. I'm just feeling really smart today because I stayed at the Holiday Inn last night." My point is that health insurance claims adjusters are making medical decisions without any medical training at all. The adjuster's job is to deny benefits or cut claims, and if he doesn't perform, he gets canned.

Economist Robert Reich recently wrote about the current state of affairs in the healthcare debate:

> So the compromise that ended up in the House bill is to have a mere public option, open only to the 6 million Americans otherwise not covered. The Congressional Budget Office warns this shrunken public option will have no real bargaining leverage and would attract mainly people who need lots of health care to begin with. So it will actually cost more than it saves.
>
> But even the House's shrunken and costly little public option is too much for private insurers, Big Pharma, Republicans and "centrists" in the Senate. So, Harry Reid has proposed an even tinier public option, which states can decide not to offer their citizens. According to the CBO, it would attract no more than four million Americans.
>
> It's a token public option, an ersatz public option, a fleeting gesture toward the idea of a public option, so small and desiccated as to be barely worth mentioning except for the fact that it still (gasp) contains the word "public."
>
> Our private, for-profit health insurance system, designed to fatten the profits of private health insurers and Big Pharma, is about to be turned over to...our private, for-profit health care system. Except that now private health insurers and Big Pharma will be getting some 30 million additional customers paid for by the rest of us.
>
> Upbeat policy wonks and political spinners who tend to see only portions of cups that are full will point out some good things: no pre-existing conditions, insurance exchanges, 30 million more

Americans covered. But in reality, the cup is 90% empty. Most of us will remain stuck with little or no choice—dependent on private insurers who care only about the bottom line, who deny our claims, who charge us more and more for co-payments and deductibles, who bury us in forms, who don't take our calls. [3]

You may be thinking, "Why is Dr. Marvin talking about economics in a book that's supposed to be about healthcare?" My answer is that you can't separate economics and politics from healthcare, not in this country anyway. Healthcare laws, like almost all other laws in this country, are unfortunately written by lobbyists. Politicians are so busy raising funds for astronomically expensive campaigns that they rely heavily on lobbyists to write legislation. That's the bottom line.

Pharmaceutical companies don't care about your health. They know they're making people sicker. It's big business! Pharmaceutical drugs are the second highest gross domestic product (GDP) every year, second only to weapons. In the U.S., pharmaceutical companies spend $19 billion a year on promotions, which include advertising, marketing, and lobbying. That's a lot of convincing. But it sure is working!

Melly Alazraki, who reports for www.DailyFinance.com regarding the extreme price increases over a period of eight years, states, "The Government Accountability Office has found that between 2000 and 2008, the prices for 321 different brand-name drugs soared from 100% to more than 2000%." [4]

The drug company Merck is a perfect example of pharmaceutical companies' lack of concern for the public's health with its recent Vioxx scandal. Mike Adams, editor of www.Natural News.com reports:

The Vioxx scandal widened this week as new research published in the Archives of Internal Medicine reveals that Vioxx maker Merck held data for three years that proved Vioxx caused an alarming increase in the risk of heart attack and strokes. And yet Merck chose not to release that data. In fact it took three more years of patients dying from heart attacks before Vioxx was pulled off the market, and even then, Merck insisted the drug was not dangerous.

This new study was based on a meta-analysis of several **unpublished studies** that Merck obviously didn't want to see published in medical journals. Drug companies routinely engage in this subterfuge: they cherry pick which studies they want published while burying the rest. They also choose which studies to forward to the FDA, all while claiming the whole charade is based on "evidence-based medicine."

It is, sort of. If you add the word "selective" in front of the phrase, making it: "Selective evidence-based medicine." [5]

An April 16, 2008 article from the *Journal of the American Medical Association* exposes the fraud of the pharmaceutical industry and its corruption of the medical profession. The article was written by the journal's Editor-in-Chief, Catherine D. DeAngelis, MD, MPH, and by Executive Deputy Editor, Phil B. Fontanarosa, MD, MBA. Drs. DeAngelis and Fontanarosa state, "The profession of medicine, in every aspect—clinical, education, and research—has been inundated with profound influence from the pharmaceutical and medical device industries. This has occurred because physicians have allowed it to happen, and it is time to stop."

Two additional articles in this same issue of *JAMA* provide a glimpse of drug company Merck's "misrepresentation of research data and its manipulation of clinical research articles and clinical reviews; such information and articles influence the education and clinical practice of physicians and other health professionals," comments Dr. Daniel Murphy, D.C. "Merck apparently manipulated dozens of publications to promote its Cox-2 inhibitor drug Vioxx. The manipulation included study results, authors, editors, and reviewers, and it only became public because of litigation involving Vioxx." [6]

Frankly, it's a breath of fresh air to see the editors of the most prestigious medical journal taking a stand, and charging medical doctors to detach themselves from the financial influence of the pharmaceutical and medical device industries. Unfortunately, doctors of integrity and influence such as DeAngelis and Fontanarosa seem to be a rare breed.

For years I wondered why the medical profession holds such influence over public health issues until I read Dr. Eleanor McBean's *The Poisoned Needle*, which cites a speech given at the annual convention of the AMA in 1911 that set the precedent. At that meeting, Dr. W.A. Evans, one of the top medical "bosses" of that time and Health Commissioner for the City of Chicago, charged his colleagues with these instructions:

> The thing for the medical profession to do, is to get right into, and man every important health movement; man health departments, tuberculosis societies, housing societies, child care and infant societies, etc. The future of the profession depends upon it...The profession cannot afford to have these places occupied by other than medical men. [7]

Some might say, "Well, that was almost a century ago." My response is, "Yes, and the medical profession has succeeded admirably well in carrying out Dr. Evans' charges. Dr. McBean comments upon this misguided crusade for power:

> This pronouncement was published in the journal of the A.M.A., September 16, 1911. Just how wholeheartedly this decree was carried out is clearly shown by how completely all the non-medical schools of healing such as chiropractic, naturopathic, religious science, hygienic, etc. have been excluded from such tax supported institutions as health boards, public hospitals, army camps, state prisons, workmen's compensation bureaus, asylums, etc. [8]

Annie Riley Hale's comments in her book *Medical Voodoo*, regarding Dr. Evans' speech are very clear in exposing his mindset:

> That the "future of his profession depended" on getting the whip-hand in Public Health Service, and that "the profession could not afford" to forgo the political advantage accruing from such monopoly will be interpreted by some as a virtual confession on the part of regular medicine that it either realized it had nothing of therapeutic value to offer the sick world, or that it had despaired of winning the sick patronage by fair means, and must therefore recourse to political intrigue.
>
> However it may be interpreted, here we have recorded evidence of a deliberate plan by organized medicine, openly declared in convention assembled, to monopolize a great public agency like the Public Health Service—affecting all the people and paid for by all the people—to the utter exclusion of all other healing professions legalized under existing laws. [9]

If you combine this deliberate political monopoly with lobbyists for the American Medical Association and pharmaceutical industry, it's easy to see that they have a vise-like grip on healthcare in the United States. Dr. McBean sheds light on the power of lobbyists over legislators by quoting from the *New York Times* of June 15, 1952:

> Some rather expert observations of the art of lobbying as practiced in Washington assert that the A.M.A. is the only organization in the country that could marshal 140 votes in Congress between sundown Friday night and noon on Monday. Performances of this sort have led some to describe the A.M.A lobby as the most powerful in the country. [10]

Dr. McBean shows that the A.M.A. even seems to have a monopoly on words.

> The word CURE has been taken over by the medical trust as its private property and drugless doctors and writers have been barred from the mails and persecuted in other ways for teaching how nature cures or for using or speaking of a cure for some disease. [11]

Anyone who has produced even a health supplement or any health product or service for that matter, cannot use the word CURE, or he will be immediately shut down. Meanwhile, the medical profession is clueless about how to cure any disease, precisely because it is totally oblivious to what is causing disease.

McBean notes that Dr. John Tilden, a medical practitioner for half a century, made the following observation, regarding inadequate medical procedures:

> Ability to cure has not kept pace with diagnosis, and today we behold the scientific paradox of skilled physicians sometimes

knowing exactly what disease the patient is suffering with, but unable to cure the disease…Ability to diagnose, but impotence in curing, is the true status of scientific medicine. [12]

As Immanuel Kant said, "Physicians think they are doing something for you by labeling what you have as a disease."

Dr. Tilden comments again:

Clinicians are floundering about in a sea of speculation and uncertainty concerning cause and cure; and the best of them declare that autopsies prove that almost half of their diagnoses are wrong. (Dr. Charles Mayo, in a radio broadcast stated that at his own clinic, autopsies showed that only 20% of diagnoses were correct.)

But the question will not (be put) down: **How is a disease to be prevented or cured when the cause is unknown?** All 400 or more so-called diseases are nothing more than expressions of our general systemic derangement—states which I am pleased to name toxemia, or healing crises. Toxemia is a state of body poisoning—self generated or induced by vaccine serums, drugs or other poisons. [13]

I'm very thankful to have skilled medical doctors available to intervene in a medical emergency or crisis. They're great at crisis care. But in my opinion, they're not so great at healthcare. I have great respect for physicians who dedicate their lives to helping the sick regain their health. The problem is not the physicians themselves, who are usually well-intentioned; the problem is that the physicians are working within a sickness care model, rather than a true healthcare model, and most of them don't realize they are being limited from effectively helping people because they themselves have been programmed by Big Medicine to work within this narrow-minded paradigm.

Let's put it this way. If your car is dehydrated (low on water), eventually it will overheat. Would you give it medication (some other chemical) to try and make it not overheat? Or would you simply add water? If your oil light were flashing (a symptom), would you add oil, or would you cover up the oil light with masking tape to cover up or mask its symptoms (the annoying blinking light)? Sound ludicrous? This is what most Americans are doing to their bodies. Our bodies may appear unintelligent, but maybe we're the ignorant ones, unaware of the body's basic needs, and our bodies are just doing the best they can with the limited resources we're giving them (such as insufficient water).

The word DOCTOR comes from the Greek term *di-daktor*, meaning "one who imparts knowledge to others—a teacher." Latin condensed the term to *doc-to-ro* and it was later shortened to "doctor." Despite the word's origins, today, medical doctors are not teachers. In fact, medical schools instruct them not to tell their patients very much. Since doctors, as a rule, are not well-informed on the real causes and cures of diseases, they could not teach their patients if they wanted to.

With this kind of "healthcare" system in place, don't you think it's a good idea to learn to take responsibility for your own health? In writing this book, I am attempting to fulfill the true role of a doctor (teacher) by giving you knowledge that can empower you to reclaim not only responsibility (for your health) but also to reclaim your health as well.

CHAPTER TWO

YOUR BODY (OF H$_2$0) AND WATER

Medical professionals do not understand the vital role of water in the human body.
— F. Batmanghelidj, M.D.

My fascination with water started as a teenager. I grew up in Hawaii, and was introduced to surfing at the age of fifteen. Actually, I would have started surfing sooner, as my best friend in the third grade was already surfing by then. But my mom, in her infinite wisdom, said "You'll just smoke pakalolo ("crazy weed" in Hawaiian, most commonly known as marijuana), get hit on the head by your surfboard and drown." Well, she was only partially right. I didn't drown. My friends would come to my house with surfboards on the racks on the car roof, and say "Let's go!" I was scared, petrified actually, so I made excuses like "I don't have a board," to which they'd respond "we've got one for you." "I don't have a leash" (a surf leash connects your board to your ankle, so you don't have to swim every time you fall off). "We've got one for you." "I have things to do at home." "Puka panty!" *Puka* means "hole" in Hawaiian, so they were basically saying, "You've got a hole in your panty, you sissy!") So I'd always end up going, and soon saw the futility in resisting. But once out at sea, what seemed to be a half mile out (but was actually more like one or two hundred yards from shore), I was completely petrified with fear! Everything looked like chaos and looming destruction to me (my destruction). That's when I first started praying to God. "Please God, just let me get back safely to shore this one last time, and I promise I'll never come out here again." Obviously God held up His/Her end of the bargain, but I didn't.

The peer pressure was too great! One day though, it was like my perception instantly cleared! All of a sudden, I saw the order and harmony to the waves. I saw how a surfer could catch a wave at point A and ride it all the way to point B. I rapidly started getting better and better at surfing. I became better at it than most of the athletic kids on my block (It seemed like half the football team lived on my block). Even better than those who had been surfing a lot longer than me. My self-confidence sky-rocketed! I was hooked! I fell in love with surfing and thought that waves were the most beautiful thing on the planet. I still do, as you can probably tell from this book's cover. Water is an amazing medium. Surfing is an incredibly rich sensual experience, to which nothing else can compare. Riding through the tube of a wave is the most physically exhilarating thing I've ever experienced. I now understand that in the tube especially is a tremendous energy field created by all the negative ions generated by the turbulent and powerful movement of water. So considering how my love of surfing is so connected to water ions, how fitting it is that ionized water should cure me of allergies!

In this chapter, we'll take a look at some of water's amazing qualities and characteristics. My intention is for you to grasp the indispensable and vital role water plays in your body, and for you to realize that simply drinking more water (especially ionized, hexagonal water) will go further to improve your health than most people realize.

Our bodies are mostly water. We're 70% water by volume, and 99% of our body's molecules are water. (The remaining 1% is comprised of bigger molecules that make up 30% of our body volume.) This beautiful planet we live on is also 70% water.

The earth contains an unimaginable 146,000,000,000,000 tons of water—that's no typo—it's 146 trillion! Deservingly, our earth is often called "the water planet." [1]

We are water beings living on a water planet. Whenever scientists are looking for life on other planets, they look for water because water is essential to all life.

When we think of essential nutrients, we commonly think of proteins, carbohydrates, fats, vitamins, and minerals. But next to oxygen, water is the MOST essential nutrient. We can survive many days (weeks) without food, but only generally three to seven days without water. Water constitutes 90% of our blood, 85% of our brain, and 75% of muscle tissue. Our body is bathed in an ocean of water and mineral salts (just like the ocean), and chemical reactions (metabolic processes) are constantly occurring at an astounding number every second. These chemical reactions require water as a medium, for water is a universal solvent, as well as a conduit for electrical current. The food we eat and the oxygen we breathe chemically combine and react to produce electricity. Water moving in and out of cells also produces electricity, by the hydroelectric effect. The electricity produced in the cells, scaled up from nanometers (the size of cells) to meters, is about the same electrical charge as that carried by the main body of a thunderstorm. That's amazing, isn't it?

Water can dissolve substances, bond with them, and transport them. It often is either involved in producing a chemical reaction, or is a product of a chemical reaction. It also can store and transfer energy within the body.

Water has many unique and special properties that make it the perfect molecule for all life to revolve around. It has a high specific heat, which simply means it can absorb a tremendous amount of heat (energy) with a minimal rise in temperature. This ability makes it very efficient at moderating temperature, which is why temperatures around large bodies of water (oceans and lakes) are more moderate. The water absorbs the heat from the sun during the day, and it radiates that heat into the atmosphere at night. Water's capacity to store so much energy makes it the perfect source for transferring energy within biological systems. [2]

Water has a very high surface tension (second in liquids only to mercury) because water molecules have a very strong attraction to each other, holding them together tightly. For this reason, water rarely (for very brief moments) appears as individual molecules. Water molecules have a very strong affinity for each other, and therefore, are almost always seen in clusters (of molecules).

Statistics regarding water levels in our body also provide a big clue about how water affects our health and the aging process. Dr. Mu Shik Jhon, a medical doctor from Korea who has done extensive research into hexagonal water, states in his book *The Water Puzzle and the Hexagonal Key*, "Infants are approximately 80% water by weight, yet it is not uncommon for the amount of water in the elderly to be below 50%." [3]

Another interesting statistic relates to cell water turnover, which simply means the amount of water discharged from the body on a daily basis. An infant in the first year of life will excrete from 125-150 ml of water per kilogram of body weight. By the time the child is a young adult that number has dropped to 25 for women and 30 for men. [4] This drop is significant because cell water turnover has been correlated with metabolic rate, and both have been linked to health and aging. Imagine how low this number must be for people in their fifties or sixties!

To illustrate the value of water's "house-cleaning" ability, let's look at an experiment performed by scientist Alexia Carrell. He kept a piece of chicken heart alive for 28 years, just by daily changing the water in the container it was in. This is pretty amazing since chickens normally do not live anywhere near 28 years; it shows the ability of cells to live indefinitely, when waste products are eliminated efficiently. In his book *Change your Water, Change Your Life*, Dr. Carpenter provides the simple analogy to our bodies of cleaning the water in a fish tank daily to keep the fish happy and healthy.

ALL WATERS ARE NOT CREATED EQUAL

Normal tap water (and even well water) has a pentagonal structure. Because of its high surface tension (water molecules have a stronger attraction for each other than for other molecules), water molecules are almost always clustered in groups of molecules. Nuclear magnetic resonance imaging has shown these pentagonal structures to have 10-13 molecules per cluster.

HEXAGONAL WATER

When water is ionized, it creates a hexagonal structure to the water molecules' cluster. Hexagonal water has been shown to contain 5-6 molecules per cluster. Among its advantages, hexagonal water improves cell water turnover. Because hexagonal units are smaller than unorganized water conglomerates, they more quickly penetrate cells, which thereby improves metabolism, nutrient absorption, and waste removal. [5] Water is absorbed into our bodies' cells as a cluster, so ionized, hexagonal water's smaller cluster size allows it to be more readily absorbed.

Hexagonal water is present in nature in only two forms: snow and glacial ice. The super cooling of water in the atmosphere creates the hexagonal structuring of snow, and consequently glacial ice. This hexagonal structure may very likely be the reason for the exceptional health and longevity of the Hunzas in the high Himalayas, as well as those living in the Caucasus Mountains of southeastern Russia, both of whom drink glacial ice water very close to its source. In addition to the water's hexagonal structure, glacial runoff also provides a high level of dissolved ions. The Japanese have had access to ionized water for over 35 years now—no wonder they rank highest in the world for health and longevity. As stated earlier, 1 in 5 households in Japan have Kangen Water™ machines (water ionizers). In Ginza, Tokyo, a city much like Manhattan, New York with its savvy Yuppies, 75-80% of households (apartments) have a Kangen Water™ machine.

Water also has the astounding capacity for memory. As Dr. Masaru Emoto shows in his amazing book *The Hidden Messages in Water*, water has the ability to be imprinted with consciousness (our thoughts) and displays itself in a form reflective of those thoughts.

Dr. Emoto concludes from his studies, "I am fully convinced that water is able to memorize and transport information; but this suggestion has been rejected by the conventional medical community." [6]

Angry and hostile thoughts imprinted into the water (by something as simple as a word written on a piece of paper and taped to the jar containing the water) show up as chaotic and disordered patterns when the water forms into crystals, whereas thoughts of love and peace appear as beautiful, symmetrical, crystalline structures.

Dr. Emoto explains how studying water crystals has provided a better understanding of water and how its state of health affects our own body's health. "The water of Tokyo was a disaster—not a single complete crystal was formed. Tap water includes a dose of chlorine, utterly destroying the structure found in natural water. However, within natural water, whether from natural springs, underground rivers, glaciers, or the upper reaches of rivers, complete crystals formed." [7]

By the same token, water "imprinted" with an electric current (as in ionized water) takes on a different structure; a hexagonal water cluster, with a higher frequency of vibration. Dr. Mu Shik Jhon likes to call hexagonal water "energized water."

Finally, hexagonal, ionized water has two other health-giving qualities. Due to its abundance of free electrons, ionized water is a powerful anti-oxidant. Secondly, ionized water can be adjusted to any pH desired. Since our bodies have a tendency toward the acidic side, drinking alkaline water can bring our body's cells and interstitial fluids (which our cells are bathed in) to a more optimal, slightly alkaline pH range (6.8-7.2). The normal pH of our blood is between 7.35 and 7.45.

Obviously, the importance of water to our bodies cannot be underestimated, and the lack of water causes serious health issues. In the following chapters, I'll discuss dehydration in more depth, including how it is responsible for many (even most) diseases.

CHAPTER THREE

CAUSES OF MOST DISEASES

The doctor of the future will give no medicine, but will interest his patients in the care of the human frame, in diet and in the cause and prevention of disease.

— **Thomas Edison**

Thomas Edison, the brilliant genius who gave us the light bulb, had a vision of what doctors should become—focusing on cause and prevention rather than treating illnesses with medications to hide the cause of pain and other symptoms. Held to Mr. Edison's standards, today's medical doctors fail in every single respect. First, all they do is give medicine. Secondly, they do not make, or even attempt to make, their patients interested in the care of the human frame—a care in which chiropractors specialize. Some of the more progressive medical doctors interest their patients in diet, but most don't bother. Finally, they certainly do not interest their patients in the cause and prevention of disease, precisely because they don't have a clue about what causes any disease. If you knew the cause of a disease, there would be no need for medications to suppress its symptoms because there usually aren't any symptoms without the disease.

In this chapter, you'll discover that a great number of ailments (even most diseases) have their roots in dehydration. You'll also learn that ionized water has additional healing and health-giving properties neither regular tap water or even well water possess. Along with dehydration, two other very common causes of disease are free radical destruction and an acidic condition in the body. You'll come to understand the interconnectedness of these three factors, and how each aggravates the others. Together, they wreak a lot of havoc in the body.

Nearly all diseases stem from either a nutrient deficiency or an excess of harmful substances in the body. I say excess because our bodies are usually able to handle and eliminate harmful substances in smaller amounts.

The most common and devastating deficiency is a deficiency of water, otherwise known as dehydration. Research says that 75% of Americans are dehydrated. I'm sure this statistic surprises many people, who run out to health food stores to find the nutrients they believe they are missing when all along, what they most need is as close as their own kitchen faucet.

Perhaps the most common and destructive substance to the human body is free radicals. You'll be amazed when you learn about the main sources of free radicals and their far reaching and destructive nature. You'll be even more surprised when you learn what an easy fix it is to defeat them.

Acidity results from a combined accumulation of harmful substances and toxins, and from the "house cleaning" functions of the body being overwhelmed (usually due to dehydration). This situation allows toxins to build up. Acidity then sets the stage, or the optimal environment, for disease to thrive.

Three causes of diseases—dehydration, free radicals, and acidity—are so common and adverse to the body's health that I will address each one individually.

My intention is to paint a clear picture in your mind of how basic functions in your body are intimately related to these three factors, and how they affect your health. By understanding the importance of these factors, you will be well on your way to taking charge of your own health, and enjoying a much healthier life.

DEHYDRATION

Dehydration is the most important and greatest cause of disease in the body. Dr. Russell Blaylock, a retired neurosurgeon, says that most people hospitalized today do not need intensive care, but rather they are hospitalized for dehydration and immediately given IV fluids. If this is true, and it's well-known that 75% of Americans are dehydrated, why in the world don't medical doctors tell people to drink more water? The answer is that it doesn't profit anyone, except the patient. If we all drank more water, there would be far fewer sick people, which would mean less business for medical doctors and the pharmaceutical industry.

Several reasons exist for the high prevalence of dehydration. One major reason is our lifestyle habit of replacing water with sodas, juices, and coffee. In his book Your Body's Many Cries for Water, Dr. Fereydoon Batmanghelidj explains how this lifestyle has been detrimental to our bodies:

> In advanced societies, thinking that tea, coffee, alcohol and manufactured beverages are desirable substitutes for the purely natural water needs of the daily "stressed" body is an elementary but catastrophic mistake. It is true that these beverages contain water, but they also contain dehydrating agents. They get rid of the water they are dissolved in plus some more water from the reserves of the body! [1]

As stated earlier, another reason for the high prevalence of dehydration is that regular water (pentagonal water) is not as easily absorbed into the body as hexagonal water. Previous generations did better with regular (pentagonal) water because they did not have as great an opportunity to indulge in dehydrating drinks as we do in modern society. The increased stress of living in modern society without the physical activity to balance it also creates a greater demand for water on the body.

Our thirst mechanism also diminishes with age. Waiting to get thirsty before drinking is not such a great idea because the sharpness of thirst perception is gradually lost as we get older. In another book, Water for Health, for Healing, for Life, Dr. Batmanghelidj states, "Phillips and associates have shown that after 24 hours of water deprivation, the elderly still do not recognize that they are thirsty. The important finding is that despite their obvious physiologic need, the elderly subjects were not markedly thirsty." [2] No wonder people are often less than 50% water by the time they die!

Dehydration and acidity are linked to and exacerbate each other. For instance, if your body is short on water, it's not likely to use much of its limited supply of water on house cleaning. Its priority will be to send the water to more vital organs (such as your brain, which you'll recall is 85% water) to keep you alive and functioning the best you can with the limited water supply. When you don't clean house very often, toxins build up and you become more acidic. Most people's bodies are in this condition.

HISTAMINE AND DEHYDRATION

When you become dehydrated, one of the first things your body does is to produce histamine. Why? Because histamine is the neurotransmitter for drought management control. It's in charge of managing a water shortage. The greater the water shortage, the more histamine the body produces.

Dr. Batmanghelidj explains, "It is scientifically clear that the histamine-directed and -operated neurotransmitter system becomes active and initiates the subordinate systems that promote water intake by triggering the thirst signals of the body." [3]

The subordinate system, which histamine uses to promote increased water intake and regulate its distribution "employs vasopressin, renin-angiotensin, prostaglandins, and kinins as intermediary agents." [4] Vasopressin and renin-angiotensin are primarily involved in regulating the distribution of water. Prostaglandins and kinins are mainly used to trigger thirst signals via pain. When these neurotransmitters come across pain sensing nerves in the body, they produce pain. The *salivary* kinins also trigger the increased production of saliva to lubricate the mouth in a dehydrated body, as well as to aid in the breakdown of food. For this reason, dry mouth is not a reliable indicator of thirst, as it usually only shows up when dehydration is more severe.

Dr. Batmanghelidj explains further:

> Pain is a sensation that denotes local chemical changes in the area around the nerves that monitor the acid/alkali balance. The mechanism is designed to safeguard against a buildup of excess acid from metabolism that could "burn" and eat into the cell membranes and the inner structures of the cells in the area. When water is not available to wash the acidic toxic waste of metabolism, the nerve endings sense the change and report it to the brain's pain centers. [5]

In other words, a slightly alkaline environment in the body is imperative for good health; acidity in the body is by itself capable of producing pain. (No wonder drinking ionized alkaline water not only relieves pain, but also provides a feeling of energy and well-being.) As we will learn later, acidity is also the breeding ground for disease. Additionally, the link between acidity and dehydration is very strong because it takes water to wash away the acidic toxic waste. This process is the same as in the colon, where copious amounts of water are required to move waste products through it.

A major implication in this mechanism of pain production is that inexplicable pain (outside of obvious injury or infection) is likely due to a water shortage. As stated earlier, most hospital admissions are due to dehydration. Imagine the numbers of dehydrated people who are not included in the statistical 75% of dehydrated Americans. I truly believe 75% is on the low side. Fibromyalgia is one of those inexplicable pains about whose cause medical doctors are clueless. Additional common effects of dehydration that Dr. Batmanghelidj lists are dyspepsia, heartburn, rheumatoid pain, back pain, angina pain (heart), headaches, and leg pain. He states, "At an early phase, the locally registered pain can be alleviated with pain killers. After a certain threshold is reached, the brain becomes the direct center for monitoring its perpetuation until hydration of the body takes place." [6]

Wow! Just think of all the innumerable people taking drugs for different types of pain when all along the "cure" was as simple as drinking more water. The worst part is that as those drugs successfully (at first) suppress the thirst symptoms of pain, the body is thrown deeper into dehydration. Dr. Batmanghelidj says that almost all pain medications cut the connection between histamine and its subordinate regulators, prostaglandins and kinins. [7]

Most of us regard histamine as an undesirable molecule our body produces that causes asthma and allergies. But the primary reason our body produces histamine is to manage a water shortage. When you become dehydrated, a side effect is that histamine causes an inflammatory response in the body (sort of like your car overheating when it's short on water), giving rise to allergies, asthma, and inexplicable chronic pain throughout the body.

Dr. Batmanghelidj highlights that the medical community misunderstands the purposes of histamine:

At present, the medical industry fraudulently and knowingly

presents histamine as a nuisance substance and produces chemical substances that interfere with and block its actions. All drugs used as pain medications, as anti-allergy medications, as anti-depressants and tranquilizers are directly and indirectly very strong anti-histamines. And yet water is an infinitely better natural antihistamine than all of them. [8]

High cholesterol is another response to dehydration. According to Dr. Batmanghelidj, it is the body's response to try and "seal off" water loss. (We'll cover high cholesterol in more depth in the chapter on heart disease, including how cholesterol has many important functions in the body, including to repair cellular damage.) So how do medical doctors handle this other symptom of dehydration? They give patients more drugs. Lipitor is advertised as the #1 prescribed branded medication in the world. Over 29 million people in the United States have been prescribed Lipitor. Again, it's big business! That's why you'll never hear about the value of cholesterol from any medical school or institution. Most medical doctors are just doing and saying what they've been taught to do and say.

Occasionally, along comes a thinking man who sees beyond the medical dogma; he rebels against the system because he cares enough about his patients to take on the monumental task of trying to revolutionize healthcare by exposing the flawed thinking and approach of our medical system. Dr. Batmanghelidj, M.D., is such a man. He has also healed many patients, who suffer from a wide variety of diseases, just by getting them to drink more water...regular water! Imagine what even greater results could be had with ionized hexagonal water!

In a more general way, dehydration (as we said earlier) decreases house cleaning, thereby increasing the toxic load on the body, and increasing acidity. In an effort to "seal off" the toxins, the body surrounds them with fat molecules to reduce the toxic effects; as a result, many people who start drinking ionized, hexagonal water experience significant weight loss. As the toxins are flushed out of the body, the fat is no longer required to isolate them from the rest of the body, so the fat is flushed out along with the toxins, or burned for energy. In a CDC study done in 2005-2006, the obesity rate for adult Americans over 20 years of age was 34%. Americans spend a lot of money on various diets and all sorts of weight loss strategies. Is it possible that drinking hexagonal water would help them to shed pounds easily and quickly? Dr. Mu Shik Jhon believes so:

> In reality, the overweight individual has a reduced amount of total body water—up to 20% less than a normal individual. Since age, metabolic rate and water structure are directly related, the fact(s) that overweight individuals have a reduced metabolic rate and a reduced amount of total body water, indicates the potential for resolve with increasing amounts of Hexagonal Water. [9]

Another place that dehydration has a big effect is in the red blood cells. Dehydration causes red blood cells to become more viscous (thicker and "stickier") and sluggish. The blood becomes more acidic. Less free oxygen is available, which then leads to fermentation, creating a breeding ground environment in which disease can flourish. This situation also likely increases the chances of plaque build-up.

Today, people spend a lot of money trying to make their skin appear youthful via cosmetic surgery, Botox, and all kinds of lotions and creams. What if aging and wrinkled skin were primarily due to dehydration? In dehydration, water is prioritized and parceled out accordingly to the more vital organs first. Guess what's low on the priority list? Furthermore, one of skin's functions is to keep water from getting in or out of the body. In light of this, doesn't it seem a bit futile trying to "moisturize" the skin? Instead, why not "moisturize" from within, by keeping the body well hydrated? Do infants look like they need moisturizer? No, because they're 80-90% water, whereas most adults are probably well under 70% water. Remember, by the time a person dies, he or she is often less than 50% water. Because your skin is low on the priority list for getting water, by the time your skin is looking like a prune, can you imagine what's going on in your more vital organs?

Some of the symptoms of mild to moderate dehydration (according to the Mayo Clinic) are:

- Dry, sticky mouth (According to Dr. Batmanghelidj, the symptom of dry mouth does not show up until the person is in a more advanced stage of dehydration).

- Thirst (Although, the thirst mechanism decreases with age, until it is almost absent in the elderly).

- Few or no tears when crying.

- Sleepiness or tiredness—children are likely to be less active than usual.

- Decreased urine output.

- Muscle weakness.

- Headache.

- Dizziness or lightheadedness.

Some of the symptoms of severe dehydration are:

- Extreme thirst.

- Very dry mouth, skin, and mucous membranes.

- Lack of sweating.

- Sunken Eyes.

- Shriveled and dry skin that lacks elasticity and doesn't "bounce back" when pinched into a fold.

- Extreme fussiness or sleepiness in infants and children; irritability and confusion in adults.

- Little or no urination—any urine that is produced will be dark yellow or amber in color.

- Low blood pressure (I believe that in mild to moderate dehydration, high blood pressure will result, as the body compensates by increasing blood pressure to "inject" water into the cells.).

- Rapid heartbeat.

- Fever.

- In the most serious cases, delirium or unconsciousness.

It's obvious from this list that dehydration (at whatever level) affects brain function. I wonder how many "mental disorders" such as depression or ADHD may be caused by something as simple as dehydration. Instead of more water being suggested, a myriad of drugs are prescribed for these "disorders."

WATER AND BRAIN FUNCTION

To understand how dehydration affects brain function, let's look at the physiology of the brain as related to water.

The brain requires a tremendous amount of energy for all its functions. It processes all the signals coming from all of the body's different parts as well as the environment (through the senses), and it responds to those signals by sending nerve impulses and neurotransmitters throughout the body. The brain never sleeps and is at work from the moment of conception to the moment of death, coordinating all the body's functions and maintaining it in a state of balance, or homeostasis. Although the brain constitutes only 1/50th of total body weight, it receives 20% of the body's blood supply.

The brain's primary sources of energy are hydroelectric energy (requiring water and salt) and sugar. In *Your Body's Many Cries for Water*, Dr. Batmanghelidj explains, "Recently it has been discovered that the human body has the ability to generate hydroelectric energy when water, by itself, goes through the cell membrane and turns some very special energy generating pumps—much like hydroelectric-power generation when a dam is built on a large river." Sugar is used not only for energy production but also for energy storage. "Storage of energy in the brain's energy pools seems to rely heavily on the availability of sugar. The brain is constantly drawing from the blood sugar to replenish its ATP and GTP stockpiles." [10] ATP (adenosine triphosphate) and GTP (guanidine triphosphate) are the body's energy storage "batteries."

Dr. Batmanghelidj then infers, "It now seems that the brain depends extensively on energy formation from hydroelectricity, particularly for its transport system in its nerve supply to different parts of the body." [11] Consequently, dehydration severely stresses the brain, especially when the body also has a salt shortage.

Additionally, Dr. Batmanghelidj adds, "It seems that dehydration *causes a severe depletion of brain tryptophan,* a most essential amino acid in the body." [12] Tryptophan is the amino acid from which serotonin, tryptamine, melatonin, and indolamine are derived. These primary neurotransmitters regulate not only brain function but also regulate all the functions of the body to maintain a state of balance, or homeostasis.

Serotonin is known as the "feel good" chemical. Medications to treat depression such as Prozac are known as SSRI's (serotonin specific re-uptake inhibitors). They inhibit the breakdown of serotonin, thus allowing higher levels of serotonin in the brain. This fact further makes me wonder about the big role dehydration might play in depression and ADHD.

ASTHMA AND ALLERGIES

I suffered with asthma at an early age. Some of my earliest memories were not pleasant ones—struggling to get enough air to breathe is a terrifying experience for anyone, let alone a four year old kid. Fortunately, I "grew out of it" within a few years. However, I soon developed allergies (asthma's wonderful cousin). You may recall that both are histamine driven. With my current understanding of physiology and medicine, I suspect that my allergies and asthma were a result not only of dehydration, but also the *routine* (at the time) childhood vaccinations. Many physicians, medical doctors as well, now know that vaccines wreak havoc on the immune system. Allergies are the body's efforts to "throw out" a foreign agent (sneezing and itchy, watery eyes). If the "invader" or foreign agent is *introduced* into the bloodstream, the poor body doesn't know what hit it, or how to deal with it. I consequently believe, as many do, that many of the auto-immune diseases have their roots in vaccinations. (I'll talk in more detail about the problems with vaccinations in a later chapter.)

Asthma causes 4,000 deaths a year in the United States (what a horrible way to go). It occurs as a chronic inflammation of the lungs in which the airways (bronchi) are reversibly narrowed. Asthma affects 7% of the population, and 300 million worldwide. During attacks (exacerbations), the smooth muscle cells in the bronchi constrict, the airways become inflamed and swollen, and breathing becomes difficult. What neurotransmitter do you suppose is responsible for causing the bronchi to constrict and the airways to become inflamed and swollen? Histamine—the very one produced by the body during a water shortage.

An allergy is an immune system disorder in which allergic reactions occur to normally harmless environmental substances known as allergens. In the U.S., 35.9 million people (or 11% of the population) suffer from allergic rhinitis. [13] Again, histamine appears to be the culprit, but the real culprit is dehydration.

DIGESTION AND DEHYDRATION

To appreciate the value and importance of water in digestion and elimination, it is necessary to understand some basic anatomy and physiology.

The stomach requires copious amounts of water, as does the pancreas for the digestive process. When water is taken in, it is absorbed into the intestines, but within half an hour, almost the same amount of water is secreted into the stomach through its glandular layer in the mucosa. (For this reason, it's a good idea to drink at least a full glass of water half an hour before meals.) This water mixes with hydrochloric acid and other enzymes to break the food down into a homogenized fluid. A mucous layer consisting of 98% water and 2% solids protects the stomach lining. The cells below the mucosal layer also secrete bicarbonate that is held in the water layer to protect further from any acid getting through the mucosal layer. The bicarbonate neutralizes any acid that tries to go through the mucosal layer. Water is also used to wash out any salts that may have accumulated in the mucosal layer during this process.

From here, the homogenized fluid mixture is released into the duodenum. It is the pancreas' job to immediately neutralize this acidic fluid by secreting large amounts of a watery bicarbonate fluid, which also requires a tremendous amount of water. If there is insufficient water for this process, the stomach will not release its contents, which can lead to heartburn, dyspepsia, and even hiatal hernia, as the body goes into reverse peristalsis from not wanting to dump the acidic mixture into an unprotected duodenum.

At this point, people suffering with heartburn or dyspepsia usually take an antacid to calm their heartburn, but again the true problem is insufficient water. Antacids add to the problem with aluminum toxicity, while the body cries out for water.

Dr. Batmanghelidj explains what happens in the digestive system during peristalsis, "When we drink water, depending on the volume of water that enters the stomach, a hormone/neurotransmitter called motilin is secreted. The more water we drink, the more motilin is produced by the intestinal tract and can be measured in blood circulation." [13] Motilin is responsible for the rhythmic contraction called peristalsis that propels the contents all the way from the upper to the lower end of the intestines. With sufficient water intake, constipation does not occur. People who suffer from constipation and its resulting diseases of colitis, diverticulitis, and even colon cancer would likely resolve their ailments if they simply drank enough water.

In a later chapter, we'll see how insufficient water in the pancreas affects diabetes. For a more detailed understanding of how dehydration affects the digestive organs (including the liver), as well as the lungs and heart, read Dr. Batmanghelidj's *Your Body's Many Cries for Water*, which provides a full and thorough understanding of dehydration's effects on all these organs.

YOUR JOINTS AND THEIR WATER NEEDS

The cartilage and discs in your joints act as a cushion and lubrication between adjacent bones, and allow smooth movement to occur between these bones. They are made mostly of water (just like the rest of your body) and collagen. In *Nourishing Traditions*, Sally Fallon and Mary Enig point out, "Collagen is the most abundant protein in the body. It is the major component of joints, cartilage, skin and connective tissue. It is responsible for the 'cushion' in joints and the suppleness in the skin, which is largely due to the amount of water it holds." [15] In order to remain healthy and function properly, your joints need two primary things: water to lubricate and bring nutrients in and waste out, and exercise or movement, to "suck" the water into the joint.

When a joint is moved through its full range of motion, a vacuum is intermittently created in the joint. This vacuum "sucks" water into the joint. Your spinal discs, for example, lose their blood supply after you reach about age 25. Subsequent to that, the only way your discs receive blood and nutrients is through movement. MRI's (magnetic resonance imaging) are used in the spine most often to determine the presence of disc herniation. Additionally, a disc's health is determined by its water content. A disc said to be "desiccated" is one that is dried up, brittle, and fragmented.

Without adequate hydration, your joints do not stand a chance at being healthy. I wonder how many joint problems have dehydration as a major causative factor?

FREE RADICAL DESTRUCTION AND ANTI-OXIDANTS

Free radicals (or oxidants) are basically unstable molecules (unstable because they are lacking or missing electrons in their outer electron shell) such as active oxygen (the unstable form of oxygen) that is looking to "steal electrons" to become stable again. When these unstable molecules come in contact with any other molecule, they steal electrons from it. This process, called oxidation, is the reason why foods such as apples and avocados turn brown when exposed to the air for a period of time. The active oxygen (which comprises 20% of oxygen) in the air steals electrons from the fruit, destroying its cells and turning it brown. A similar destructive process happens in the body when it is exposed to free radicals.

The body produces free radicals by normal metabolic processes, but their production is accelerated by stress (physical, mental/emotional, or chemical). Physical stress is produced by strenuous physical activity such as exercise or hard labor. Chemical stress is caused by chemicals in food or drinks, or the air one breathes in the city. Mental/emotional stress is a common thing in modern life caused by constant demands for efficiency and a higher pace of living. These free radicals steal electrons from your body's cells, thereby causing destruction of those cells, which then turn into free radicals themselves, because now they too are lacking and seeking to steal other cells' electrons, thus creating a continual domino effect. No wonder anti-oxidants are the #1 selling health supplement product in the U.S.

Anti-oxidants vary in their effectiveness by their ability to provide readily available electrons, in order to donate them to stabilize the free radical molecule. Most anti-oxidants, such as Vitamins C and E or superoxide dismutase, work by being oxidized themselves. Ionized water on the other hand, works by simply donating its abundance of free electrons.

A molecule's anti-oxidant value is measured by its (-) ORP

(oxidation reduction potential) value. A high (-) ORP value indicates a strong anti-oxidant capacity. A molecule with a (+) ORP is called a free radical. A high (+) ORP is a powerful free radical. As a comparison green tea, often touted as a strong anti-oxidant, has an ORP value of -100mV (millivolts). Kangen Water™ has an ORP value of -300 to -800mV, depending on the source water.

In 2006, the global bottled water market was valued at $60,938.1 million. In 2011, the market value is forecast to reach $86,421.2 million, an increase of 41.6% in just five years. What are people getting for all that money spent? They are getting acidic water (most bottled waters test out on the acidic side) with an ORP value between +150 and +300 mV (acidic, free radical water in a bottle). Tap water can have an ORP as high as +500 mV, making it a powerful free radical. But at least it's free!

Interestingly, a direct correlation exists between ORP and pH. As pH goes up (more alkaline), the ORP increases in its (-) value. It becomes a more powerful anti-oxidant. As pH goes down (more acidic), the ORP increases in its (+) value. It becomes a more powerful free radical.

ACIDITY

A lot of misinformation and confusion surrounds pH and acid/alkaline balance in the body. In order to clear up the confusion, we first need a bit of basic chemistry and physiology. The acidity or alkalinity of a solution is measured on a scale of values called pH (parts hydrogen). The values on the pH scale range from 0 to 14, with 0 indicating the most acidic level and 14 the most alkaline.

A solution with a pH of 7 is neutral because it contains the same amount of H+ ions and OH- ions.

Many people believe our bodies should be very alkaline, when in fact most body fluids' pH should be just above neutral in general. Our intracellular (inside of cells) and extracellular (the fluid our cells are bathed in) fluids have a normal range of pH 6.8 to 7.2. The normal range of blood is even narrower, at 7.30 to 7.45.

The reason alkalinity is so strongly promoted and stressed is simply because Americans in general are so acidic! The culprit behind this situation is our Standard American Diet (S.A.D.—a fitting acronym), which is loaded with acid forming foods. Americans consume 150 pounds of refined sugar every year, 30 times more sugar than our grandparents consumed (5 pounds per year)! In addition to containing an incredible amount of "empty" (empty of nutrients) calories, sugar depletes the alkaline minerals in our body that are used to neutralize the acidity.

A diet high in sugar, meat, alcohol, dairy products, fried foods, and processed foods (such as pastas, white bread, and white rice, just to name a few) is very acid forming. As a result, when food is "burned" (or digested), the waste products left over are acidic. The average American eats 248 pounds of meat per year. Years ago, I heard that a diet high in meat increased the chances of osteoporosis. At the time I didn't understand why. Now it's more commonly known that the acidity produced by eating a lot of meat pulls calcium and other alkaline minerals out of the bones to neutralize the acidity. Dairy products are also very acid forming. The average American drinks 18 gallons of milk and eats 12 pounds of cheese and 1.5 pounds of butter in a year. The dairy industry tells people to drink lots of milk for strong and healthy bones and teeth, yet milk is actually causing osteoporosis due to its acidifying effect. I believe the reason dairy products are so acidic is because they have been pasteurized. Pasteurization uses very high heat to "sterilize" the milk.

In *Nourishing Traditions*, Fallon and Enig explain, "Pasteurization destroys all the enzymes in milk—in fact, the test for successful pasteurization is absence of enzymes. These enzymes help the body assimilate all body-building factors, including calcium." [15]

Actually, pasteurization either destroys most vitamins, minerals, proteins, and other nutrients, or it makes them less digestible or less available. It promotes rancidity of unsaturated fats with its high heat processing. In essence, most of milk's life-giving properties are stripped, destroyed, or altered by pasteurization.

Fried foods are not only very acidic, but they are also loaded with free radicals. Processed foods such as potato chips, cookies, white bread, white rice, pasta, hot dogs (the list goes on and on) are not only quite acidic, but they also sit in your colon and ferment.

One of the worst things a person can consume is soda. A can of Coca-Cola has a pH of 2.5. On top of that, the high sugar content in soda (8-12 teaspoons per can) further depletes the body of alkaline minerals because they are used up to process and excrete the sugar from the body, thereby making the body even more acidic. Most sodas range in pH from 2.5 to 4.0. And yet, Americans (and especially teenagers) guzzle 53 gallons of soda per year. It takes 32 glasses of alkaline water to neutralize the acidity produced from drinking one can of Coke! One health professional I know feels that drinking a can of soda is worse than smoking a cigarette. I understand why. Most Americans are totally oblivious to the harm done by drinking one can of soda. The problem is that the effects of drinking soda are not immediately apparent, especially when a person is young. But in effect, it's like drinking tasty poison with a temporary sugar and caffeine high. In addition to the acidity, this surge in blood sugar and caffeine is followed by an increased production of insulin to stabilize blood sugar levels. Eventually, the pancreas becomes depleted of insulin, leading to diabetes.

Our bodies function within a very narrow range of pH. When pH becomes more acidic, the 4,000 or so normal chemical reactions (metabolic processes) involving proteins and enzymes don't function properly. Proteins become denatured (structurally degraded) and devitalized. Normal metabolic processes at the cellular level suffer.

Your blood, which functions within a very narrow range of pH (7.30 to 7.45), is very sensitive to changes in pH. Your body works to keep pH alkaline by pulling alkaline minerals from your bones, organs, and wherever it can find those minerals. For this reason, people become osteoporotic with a diet high in acid-forming foods, such as meat and dairy products. It seems counter-intuitive for dairy products to cause osteoporosis because of their high calcium content, but the acid-forming nature of dairy products requires more calcium (and other alkaline minerals) to neutralize acidity than is found in the dairy product itself.

It's been found that blood at a pH of 7.45 contains 65% more excess oxygen than blood at a pH of 7.30. Why is this fact significant?

In 1931, Dr. Otto Warburg won the Nobel Prize for discovering the "cause" of cancer. He discovered that cancer can only grow in an environment with a relative absence of oxygen. In an oxygen deficient environment, the cells switch from an aerobic form of energy production to an anaerobic (no oxygen) form of fermentation of sugar. This environment allows cancer to thrive. Cancer cells are a lot like plant cells; they breathe in CO_2 and expel O_2 as a waste product. What Dr. Warburg "missed" is the cause of the oxygen deficient environment...acidity. The Japanese have known about acidity for a while, so they have reduced acidity by eating an alkaline diet and drinking alkaline water. One of the first things done in a Japanese hospital is to test the patient's pH.

Dehydration, free radicals, and acidity account for a great majority of diseases' causes. As we have seen, they are also inter-related—one condition aggravating one or both of the others. A well-hydrated, alkaline body with a minimal amount of free radicals is essential to good health. If this understanding is the only thing you get out of this book, and you apply this knowledge, your health is certain to improve.

CHAPTER FOUR

THE REMEDY

Ionized water...the Magic Elixir

CAUSES OF DISEASES AND IONIZED WATER

As stated in the previous chapter, the root causes of most diseases are dehydration, free radical destruction, and acidity. The amazing thing about ionized hexagonal water is that it addresses all three of the above in a big way. In this chapter, we'll see how ionized water has so many beneficial effects in the body, and how it works to resolve and prevent many chronic degenerative diseases.

Ionized water's hexagonal structure allows greater absorption into the cells, thereby hydrating the body like regular water never did. People who drink this water comment on how "silky" it feels going down and how it does not give them a bloated feeling when drinking more than one glass at a time (as regular water does).

• Hexagonal water is also more energetically powerful, so it really goes to town with the house cleaning. Because it passes in and out of cells easily, it also pulls toxins and waste products out of cells better than any other "cleanse" on the market. After all, water itself is the greatest solvent and transporter of waste products (and nutrients) in existence, and ionized hexagonal water is the best of the best at house cleaning. The colon provides the best evidence for ionized hexagonal water's amazing power.

THE COLON CONNECTION

The colon seems to be a mirror for the rest of the body's health. In Japan, Dr. Hiromi Shinya is known for having invented the procedure and equipment for colonoscopy. Since then, we've had the ability to get a detailed look into the colon's health condition. What becomes obvious in looking at numerous colonoscopies is the correlation between the colon's health (and cleanliness) and the body's general health. The sicker the patient (cancer, diabetes, etc.), the worse the colon looks. People with chronic, advanced degenerative diseases almost always have a colon that literally looks like a backed up sewer. What's more amazing is that as patients start to drink Kangen Water™ (ionized hexagonal water), not only do their colons change from looking like filthy sewer systems to clean, pink, spotless colons, but their overall health also improves in dramatic fashion. This transformation gives total credence to the understanding that an overly acidic condition in the body is the breeding ground for disease of all kinds. Again, ionized water provides a double whammy of benefits here. Its ability to pull waste products out of cells and dispose of them is unsurpassed. Its alkalinity neutralizes any acidic condition better than the strictest vegetarian alkaline diet, and we all know how difficult it is to sustain a diet—especially a vegetarian alkaline one. The negative ORP of ionized alkaline water also provides a benefit to the intestinal walls. In his book *Change Your Water, Change Your Life*, Dr. Dave Carpenter explains more about negative ORP:

> Bacterial microorganisms are known to flourish at different oxidation-reduction potentials (ORP). The "friendly" bacteria in the intestines are over 95% anaerobic. They require negative ORP values to flourish. Drinking water and consuming foods with a high negative ORP value supports the growth of the beneficial bacteria in the intestinal tract and helps establish ongoing microbial balance. Perhaps this is the reason that many digestive problems resolve when people begin to drink Kangen Water™. [1]

WATER AND DNA

One of water's functions in the body is to surround, stabilize, and protect DNA. Studies performed by Dr. Mu Shik Jhon and others found "that the water surrounding normal DNA is highly structured, and much less mobile than the water around abnormal DNA. This tightly-held and highly structured water which surrounds normal DNA acts to stabilize the helical structure of the DNA. It forms a layer of protection from all outside influences which could cause malfunction or distortion." [2] This highly structured, less mobile water is hexagonal water. Pentagonal water (regular water), by contrast, is less structured and more mobile. It is less stabilizing and less protective. Dr. Jhon also did a study to determine the effects of Hexagonal Water (structured water) on cultured cancer cells. "In unprocessed (pentagonal) water, tumor cells increased to 3.2 million in four days. However, the tumor cells that were exposed to alkaline ionized water (hexagonal) decreased to 20,000 during the same 4-day period." [3] Along with cancer, the study found that the water surrounding DNA in diabetic cells was also less structured and more mobile.

SUMMARY

Ionized hexagonal water hydrates the body much better than regular water, thus alleviating the problem of chronic dehydration from which so many Americans suffer. An interconnection exists between dehydration and acidity in the body. This acidity is compounded by the Standard American Diet (S.A.D.). Ionized alkaline water is the simplest and most effective solution to both of these issues. Additionally, free radical destruction can be stopped in its tracks via the high negative ORP present in ionized, alkaline, hexagonal water. Ionized water provides an abundance of free electrons to donate to the electron-hungry free radicals, thereby neutralizing them.

The body experiences certain side effects, or more specifically, cleansing reactions from drinking ionized water. First, when given sufficient alkaline water that is absorbed well, the body hydrates cells that have previously lacked sufficient water. Next, it will likely go into house cleaning mode, known as a cleansing reaction. These reactions can vary from heartburn to headaches and even constipation. Some people may even experience an increased thirst for water (even dryness in the mouth) as the body says, "Yes, give me more!"

At this point, many people mistakenly think water is making them worse. But these symptoms are temporary as the body starts to cleanse itself of long accumulated toxins and acidity, and it hydrates the body's cells that have long gone with insufficient water. If allowed to continue hydrating and cleansing, by being given more water, the body will begin to manifest health like it hasn't experienced in many years.

One more thing about ionized, hexagonal water: In the last two chapters, I hit on the most common disease conditions helped by it. However, simply because I did not mention a certain disease process does not mean it wouldn't benefit greatly from this water. Water is such a basic part of cell structure and function that any healthy or unhealthy condition would be improved with its use. Ionized water's hydrating qualities, alkalizing properties, and anti-oxidant properties provide the remedy for most disease processes, and enhance an already healthy condition. It truly is a magic elixir!

QUESTIONS AND ANSWERS

Q. What about stomach pH? Won't alkaline water neutralize the acidity of the stomach, thereby ruining digestion?

A. To the contrary, water is absolutely necessary for digestion, if taken 30 minutes prior to eating. One should also wait 2 hours after meals before drinking water. Small amounts of water (4 ounces) can be taken with meals.

Q. How much water should a person drink every day?

A. Many health experts agree that a person should drink about half of his or her body weight (lbs.) in ounces. So a 200 pound man should drink 100 ounces of water a day. (A gallon is 128 ounces).

Q. I get my "water" by drinking a lot of other beverages. Do I still need to drink that much water?

A. Drinking other beverages is not the same as drinking plain water. In fact, caffeinated and alcoholic beverages are incredibly dehydrating. Drinking these beverages actually increases the amount of water you'll need to drink. The next time you consume a fair amount of wine or another alcoholic beverage, drink a fair amount of water with it, and just see how much better you feel the next morning!

Q. Is it common to have cleansing reactions?

A. Everybody's body is different and will react differently. The healthier you are generally, the less likely you are to have cleansing reactions. If your body is loaded with toxins, acidity, and wastes, the more likely it is for you to experience a cleansing reaction. A cleansing reaction occurs as your body is pulling waste products out of the cells for disposal from the body. If excessive amounts of waste products and toxins are in your blood at one time, you will have a cleansing reaction. Fortunately, the rate at which you cleanse can be controlled by the pH of the water you drink. People who are new to drinking ionized alkaline water should start with pH 8.5 water. Most people will not have a cleansing reaction if they start at this pH.

Q. What if I'm taking medications? Is it safe to drink ionized water?

A. Ionized hexagonal water will increase the absorption of everything else you consume. In the case of supplements and even the nutrients from food in general, this increased absorption will work in your favor. In the case of medications, it will increase the rapidity of absorption and could therefore necessitate adjusting your dosage. Generally, medication should be taken an hour before or after drinking ionized water because of the increased absorption rate. Ideally, you should consult with your physician about adjusting dosages and the length of time between taking your medication and drinking ionized water. Many water ionizer systems also have a neutral 7.0 water that can be used with taking medications.

Q. Are there other uses for ionized water?

A. Yes, some water ionizers can produce strongly alkaline (11.5 pH) and strongly acidic (2.5 pH) water. One is great for cleaning (11.5), as it emulsifies fats and oils, and generally gets into fabrics and even more solid surfaces and pulls dirt and grime out of materials, just as the 8.5-9.5 water cleans out your body. One or two quarts of this strong alkaline water added to your laundry will make for much cleaner clothes. The 2.5 pH water is a powerful antiseptic. It will kill almost all bacteria and viruses on contact within 30 seconds. The applications of this acidic water are astounding. The Japanese have used this water (2.5 pH) successfully to treat gangrene. Japanese farmers spray this water on crops to protect them from microbial infestation, relieving them of the need to use harsh, toxic chemicals.

Q. What about distilled water and reverse osmosis water?

A. The Japanese consider distilled water "dead water" because all the life-giving minerals dissolved in the water are pulled out along with the undesirable toxic minerals or microorganisms. Worse yet, when in the body, this water pulls its missing minerals out of the body, causing the body to become deficient in minerals. Reverse osmosis water does pretty much the same thing. The bottom line is: **Do not drink distilled water. It's bad for your health.**

Q. What about chlorine and other chemicals present in tap water?

A. Many of these chemicals, chlorine and fluoride in particular, have damaging toxic effects in the body. Most water ionizers have a built-in filter to remove these toxins, but may not get it all out. Testing your water to ensure all of these chemical toxins have been removed is probably a good idea. An additional water filter may be needed to provide clean, chemical free water.

Q. Can a person drink too much water?

A. The answer is "Yes." Remember that a balance exists between water inside of the cells and water outside of the cells. This balance is maintained by the "salts" inside the cells (mainly potassium) and outside of the cells (primarily sodium). An excess of water can throw this balance off, just as a deficiency can. In current society though, most people lean more toward a deficiency.

CHAPTER FIVE

HEART DISEASE

Tell me lies; tell me sweet little lies…
— **Fleetwood Mac**

Heart disease is a perfect example of the medical profession's mismanagement of diseases. The problem is compounded by the incorrect information (that's the nice way of putting it) propagated by the pharmaceutical industry, the American Heart Association, the media, and even the food industry. In this chapter, we'll explore the truth behind cholesterol and saturated fats, and we'll discover the true cause of heart disease.

Heart disease or cardiopathy is an umbrella term for a variety of different diseases affecting the heart. As of 2007, heart disease is the leading cause of death in the United States, England, Canada, and Wales, killing one person every 34 seconds in the United States alone.

What are the culprits in this major killer? Are they cholesterol and saturated fats?

What does conventional medical wisdom have to say about the causes of heart disease?

INFLAMMATION

Dr. Peter Libby is an expert in the field of heart disease. He is the chief of cardiovascular medicine at Brigham and Women's Hospital, Mallinkrodt Professor of Medicine at Harvard Medical School, and co-editor of *Heart Disease,* a classic cardiology textbook. In an excellent article he wrote for *Scientific American,* Dr. Libby states:

> Only a decade ago, most physicians would have confidently described atherosclerosis as a plumbing problem: Fat-laden gunk gradually builds up on artery walls. If a deposit (plaque) grows large enough, it closes off an affected "pipe" preventing blood flow. Eventually, the blood-starved tissue dies. If that happens in the heart or the brain, a heart attack or stroke occurs. Few believe that tidy explanation anymore. Twenty years of research show that arteries bear little resemblance to pipes. They contain living cells that communicate with one another and their environment. They also participate in the fatty deposits that grow within vessel walls—few which actually shrink vessels to a pinpoint. Most heart attacks and many strokes stem from interior plaques that rupture suddenly, spawning a blood clot that blocks blood flow. *Such research has established <u>inflammation's key role in atherosclerosis.</u>* [1]

Inflammation plays a key role in both the growth of plaques and their rupture. Inflammation is produced in the arteries in two primary ways, both involving free radicals. Microbial invasion is one of the ways that free radicals are produced. I will summarize how microbial invasion works as explained by Dr. Peter Libby and Kaumudi Joshipura, Director of the Division of Dental Public Health in Puerto Rico. We'll get into the other cause of free radical production later, but the bottom line is the medical profession (including Dr. Libby) does not understand this mechanism.

When our body perceives a microbial invasion, it mobilizes its defenses—the immune system's frontline warriors, which are certain types of white blood cells that secrete chemicals to limit infection. These chemicals include oxidants (free radicals) which are meant to help destroy invading microbes, but invariably create a lot of "friendly fire." All in all, it's a pitched battle on a microscopic level. This battle produces a LOT of inflammation.

This inflammation is the reason periodontal disease has been said to increase the risk of heart disease. One of several things heart disease and periodontal disease have in common is inflammation, "which both narrows coronary arteries and breaks down the tissues that hold teeth in place. Periodontal bacteria are found in the plaque deposits that narrow coronary arteries; inducing periodontal disease in rabbits causes plaque accumulations in the coronary arteries." [2]

Let's briefly re-cap. As Dr. Libby says, research clearly shows that inflammation is at the root of heart disease, and that free radicals are responsible for this inflammation. In the previous paragraph by

Kaumudi Joshipura, we understood that one way free radicals are produced in the body, and arterial walls specifically, is in response to a perceived microbial invasion. Beyond this (a microbial threat), the medical profession is unsure what produces the free radicals that cause inflammation, leading to plaque build-up.

By now, you're probably wondering what inflammation has to do with saturated fats and cholesterol. Are saturated fats and cholesterol responsible for producing the free radicals that result in inflammation? Remember, Dr. Libby, a well-respected cardiologist, has said that inflammation is at the root of plaque build-up. He says nothing implicating saturated fats or cholesterol, however.

SATURATED FATS

So how do cholesterol and saturated fats fit into all of this? As I mentioned in the Introduction, heart disease was a rare thing before 1920.

Today, heart disease causes at least 40% of all U.S. deaths. During the sixty-year period from 1910 to 1970, the proportion of traditional animal fat in the American diet declined from 83% to 62% (of all fats consumed), and butter consumption plummeted from 18 pounds per person per year to 4 pounds. (You may recall it's now down to 1.5 pounds.) During the same period, the percentage of dietary vegetable oils in the form of margarine, shortening, and refined oils increased about 400% while the consumption of sugar and processed foods increased about 60%. [3]

This change in eating habits is largely due to what we've been told by "health experts" in the media. The health experts from the American Heart Association and the rest of the mainstream media have told us that saturated fats and cholesterol, typically from animal fats, are the bad guys, while they have touted polyunsaturated oils as "heart healthy" oils. How did they come up with this belief? **Nothing** in the research literature supports this view.

Statistics seem to show that the opposite is true. As the consumption of animal fats (primary sources of saturated fats and cholesterol) has declined significantly, and the consumption of polyunsaturated and hydrogenated oils have skyrocketed, heart disease has become our nation's biggest killer. What a coincidence!

This contradiction is confusing. We're being told to avoid cholesterol and saturated fats like the plague, while statistics show an inverse relationship between the consumption of animal fats and heart disease.

We've looked at what some of the statistics say, so now let's take a look at the science of physiology. As Dr. Batmanghelidj said about physiology in relation to histamine, "If we look at histamine within its role as a water regulator of the body, the entire structure of medicine will change and become people-friendly; and *the science of physiology will take over*." [4]

So let's look at the physiology behind cholesterol and saturated fats to see whether it will shed any light on the issue.

The book *Nourishing Traditions*, compiled by nutritionist Sally Fallon and Mary G. Enig, Ph.D., an expert of international renown in the field of lipid (fat) chemistry, begins with 70 information-packed pages on nutrition and scientific understanding, followed by healthful (and delicious) traditional recipes for the reader to put a healthy diet into practice. Here are some excerpts from *Nourishing Traditions* regarding saturated fats and cholesterol:

> The demonized saturated fats—which many Americans are trying to avoid—are not the cause of our modern diseases. In fact, they play many important roles in the body chemistry:
>
> • Saturated fatty acids constitute at least 50 percent of the cell membranes, giving them necessary stiffness and integrity so they can function properly.

How can it be that a substance that constitutes at least 50% of the cell membranes (and we're talking about every single one of the several trillion cells in your body) is the bad guy? Does that sound crazy to anybody besides me?

> • They are needed for the proper utilization of essential fatty acids. Elongated omega-3 fatty acids are better retained in the tissues when the diet is rich in saturated fats.

Well, since omega-3 fatty acids are commonly known to be heart-healthy, this fact has got to be a good thing too.

> • The heart prefers to be surrounded with saturated fats and draws on this fat reserve in times of stress. Saturated 18-carbon stearic acid and 16-carbon palmitic acid (from animal sources) provides these saturated fats.

The scientific evidence, honestly evaluated, does not support the assertion that "artery-clogging" saturated fats cause heart disease. Actually, evaluation of the fat in artery clogs reveals that only about 26 percent is saturated. The rest is unsaturated, of which more than half is polyunsaturated. [5]

This information goes hand in hand with the statistics shown earlier, implicating polyunsaturated oils and hydrogenated fats in heart disease, rather than saturated fats and cholesterol.

CHOLESTEROL

What about cholesterol? Understanding cholesterol is a little trickier. To understand it truly, we once again need to review some physiology. So stay with me—it's actually fascinating.

The name cholesterol originates from the Greek *chole-* (bile) and *stereos-* (solid), and the chemical suffix *-ol* for an alcohol. Its important roles in the body include:

- Cholesterol constitutes an essential structural component of cell membranes in all mammals. Along with saturated fats, cholesterol in the cell membranes gives our cells necessary stiffness and stability.

- It regulates membrane fluidity; in other words, what is allowed to pass through the cell membrane.

- "Cholesterol is needed for proper function of serotonin receptors in the brain. Serotonin is the body's natural 'feel good' chemical. Low cholesterol levels have been linked to aggressive and violent behavior, depression and suicidal tendencies." [6]

- Cholesterol, within the cell membrane, also plays a role in intracellular transport, cell signaling and nerve conduction. In many neurons, a myelin sheath (the covering around the nerve), rich in cholesterol, provides insulation for more efficient conduction of impulses.

- "Mother's milk is especially rich in cholesterol and contains a special enzyme that helps the baby utilize this nutrient. Babies and children need cholesterol-rich foods throughout their growing years to ensure proper development of the brain and nervous system." [7]

- In the liver, cholesterol is converted to bile, which is then stored in the gall bladder. Bile contains bile salts, which solubilize (dissolve and break down into parts) fats in the digestive tract and aid in the intestinal absorption of fat molecules as well as the fat-soluble vitamins, Vitamin A, Vitamin D, Vitamin E, and Vitamin K.

- Cholesterol also acts as an anti-oxidant, protecting against the free radical damage that leads to heart disease.

- Cholesterol is an important precursor molecule for the synthesis of Vitamin D and the steroid hormones (that help us deal with stress), including the adrenal gland hormones cortisol and aldosterone, as well as the sex hormones progesterone, estrogens, and testosterone, and their derivatives. Vitamin D is "a vital fat-soluble vitamin needed for healthy bones and nervous system, proper growth, mineral metabolism, muscle tone, insulin production, reproduction and immune system function." [8]

So with all the vital roles and functions played by cholesterol, why is it considered such a bad guy? The authors of *Nourishing Traditions* say that blaming cholesterol for heart disease is like blaming the police force for crime in a high crime area, when they are trying to prevent it.

POLYUNSATURATED OILS

Again, we come back to Dr. Libby's assertion that inflammation is at the root of coronary heart disease and free radical destruction is the number one cause of inflammation. So what causes the free radicals that lead to inflammation? "When the diet contains an excess of polyunsaturated fatty acids, these replace saturated fatty acids in the cell membrane, so that the cell walls actually become flabby."[9] In addition, these polyunsaturated oils have often already become free radicals even before being ingested into the body, due to the high heat processing of, and cooking with, these oils. Fallon and Enig explain further:

One reason the polyunsaturates cause so many health problems is that they tend to become oxidized or rancid when subjected to heat, oxygen, and moisture as in cooking and processing. Rancid oils are characterized by free radicals—that is, single atoms or clusters with an unpaired electron in an outer orbit. These chemicals are extremely reactive chemically. They have been characterized as "marauders" in the body for they attack cell membranes and red blood cells, causing damage in DNA/RNA strands that can trigger mutations in tissue, blood vessels and skin. [10]

Once these free radical oils are incorporated into the cell walls, they become destructive agents from within. Once again, the authors of *Nourishing Traditions* state:

> Our blood vessels can become damaged in a number of ways—through irritations caused by free radicals or viruses, or because they are structurally weak—and when this happens, the body's natural healing substance steps in to repair the damage. That substance is cholesterol. [11]

HDL AND LDL—GOOD VS. BAD?

At this point, I want to clear up some confusion surrounding LDL and HDL "cholesterol". I have cholesterol in quotes, because these are not really forms of cholesterol (as we've been told). LDL and HDL are actually lipoproteins (made of fat and protein) that act as carrier molecules for cholesterol in the blood stream. Since cholesterol is insoluble in blood, it is transported in the circulatory system within lipoproteins, whose outward-facing surfaces are water-soluble and inward-facing surfaces are lipid-soluble. There are several types of lipoproteins characterized by names related to their density. Low-density lipoproteins (LDL) have more fat and less protein than HDL, making them less dense. In addition to providing a soluble means for transporting cholesterol and other fats through the bloodstream, lipoproteins have cell-targeting signals that direct the lipids they carry to certain tissues.

The key points here are: 1) lipoproteins are just carrier molecules for cholesterol and other fats; 2) these lipoproteins have cell-targeting signals that direct the lipids they carry to certain tissues. In other words, LDLs are not the "bad guy" either. They are just following directions to transport cholesterol to a pre-determined location, which was likely pre-determined by the need for cholesterol as a repair substance.

The authors of *Nourishing Traditions* sum up cholesterol by saying:

> Cholesterol is not the cause of heart disease but rather a potent anti-oxidant weapon against free radicals in the blood, and a repair substance that heals arterial damage (although the arterial plaques themselves contain very little cholesterol)....However, like fats, cholesterol may be damaged by exposure to heat and oxygen. This damaged or oxidized cholesterol seems to promote both injuries to the arterial cells as well as pathological build-up of plaque in the arteries. Damaged cholesterol is found in powdered eggs, in powdered milk (added to reduced fat milks to give them body) and in meats and fats that have been heated to high temperatures in frying and other high temperature processes. [12]

(Note that the foods containing damaged cholesterol are all processed foods or foods exposed to high temperatures).

THE REAL CULPRITS

It appears that the "real culprits" here are **polyunsaturated oils and hydrogenated fats**, the very items touted as being "heart-healthy" by the American Heart Association and the mainstream media. Consider this—if this truth became common knowledge, the American Heart Association would cease to exist. Once the real cause of heart disease was widely known, the American Heart Association would serve no purpose. Crime solved; case closed.

Unfortunately, you can't separate politics from economics. The food industry would also lose out because cheap polyunsaturated oils and hydrogenated fats with their long shelf life would be avoided like the plague by informed consumers. The pharmaceutical companies would certainly take a big financial hit because no one would take Lipitor anymore. Why take Lipitor to lower cholesterol levels when cholesterol is not the problem?

Dr. Batmanghelidj gives us a slightly different view regarding cholesterol that relates back to dehydration. The cell membrane is composed of two layers, separated by a waterway for enzyme activity. Each layer has hydrocarbon bricks to give it structural integrity. Adhesive sheets of water hold these bricks together and water also diffuses through the bricks. In dehydration the waterway closes down, stopping enzyme movement. Cholesterol is a natural clay that the body uses to seal off water loss and stick the hydrocarbon bricks together. Both views see cholesterol as a repair substance, and not as the cause of atherosclerotic plaques.

In a later chapter on vaccinations, I'll discuss how vaccines are known to play a part in heart disease. In the same way that periodontal disease leads to free radical production by the immune system, a constant, looming microbial threat from vaccination would likely produce similar results.

CHAPTER SIX

DIABETES AND HIGH BLOOD PRESSURE

The...patient should be made to understand that he or she must take charge of his own life. Don't take your body to the doctor as if he were a repair shop.

— Quentin Regestein

This chapter further illustrates medical mismanagement of disease. This mismanagement becomes crystal clear when you understand normal physiology and pathophysiology (how disease is established). Both issues can either be significantly mitigated or resolved with proper dietary habits, which will be explained specifically. While reading, always think to yourself, "What's causing the body to do this?" There's a reason blood sugar levels may be high. There's a reason blood pressure may be elevated. Rather than suppressing these symptoms with medication, wouldn't you rather address the symptoms' cause?

DIABETES

Diabetes mellitus, commonly referred to as just **diabetes**—is a condition where the body either does not produce enough or does not properly respond to insulin. Insulin is a hormone produced in the pancreas that allows cells to absorb glucose for the purpose of turning it into energy. When a person has diabetes, his body either is failing to respond appropriately to its own insulin, and/or it does not make enough insulin. Either situation causes glucose accumulation in the blood, resulting in any of various complications. [1]

An estimated 23.6 million people in the U.S. (7.8% of the population) have diabetes, of which 17.9 million have been diagnosed. Of those people diagnosed, 90% of them are type 2. With prevalence rates doubling between 1990 and 2005, the CDC (Centers for Disease Control) has characterized the increase as an epidemic.

While type 2 diabetes is frequently a disease associated with adults, more and more children are being diagnosed as type 2 diabetics in parallel with the rise in obesity rates, which can be directly linked to changes in lifestyle and dietary patterns stemming from childhood. [2]

Insulin resistance or reduced insulin sensitivity results in type 2 diabetes mellitus. While type 2 is usually marked by high insulin levels, sometimes abnormally reduced insulin secretion occurs that occasionally even becomes absolute. When body tissues are defective in responding to insulin, they usually involve insulin receptors in

100

cell membranes. Cortisol, the primary hormone involved in diabetes mellitus type 2, is a stress hormone secreted by the adrenal glands. It's interesting to note that as cortisol increases (with stress), the number of insulin receptors decreases. This example reflects how mental stress affects and manifests in the body. [3]

Outside of mental stress, two major factors cause diabetes, as previously stated: decreased insulin production and decreased insulin sensitivity. But what causes decreased insulin production and sensitivity? I believe the answer is twofold: dehydration, and excessive consumption of simple carbohydrates (refined carbohydrates), respectively.

DEHYDRATION AND DIABETES

To understand the relationship between dehydration and diabetes, we need to go back to physiology. As was discussed earlier, digestion requires copious amounts of water. Before the stomach releases its acidic contents (food/fluid mixture) into the duodenum, it needs to be assured that the pancreas has secreted a sufficient amount of watery bicarbonate solution to neutralize the acidic stomach contents. When a state of dehydration is present, an insufficient amount of water is available to produce this watery bicarbonate solution. Consequently, the stomach "senses" this lack of neutralizing bicarbonate solution and holds on to its acidic contents.

The pancreas, meanwhile, has two major functions that work in opposition. Just as the sympathetic and parasympathetic nervous systems work in opposition (when the activity of one increases, the activity of the other decreases, and vice versa), it's the same with the pancreas. These two primary functions of the pancreas are: the production of this watery bicarbonate solution to neutralize stomach acid, and the production and secretion of insulin to lower blood sugar by pushing glucose into the cells. Guess which one takes priority? If you guessed the watery bicarbonate solution, you're a genius (you're correct). In other words, in a state of dehydration, the production of insulin is decreased or shut down.

REFINED CARBOHYDRATES AND DIABETES

The dietary habits of modern Americans continue to trend away from whole foods, and move toward the highly processed, refined foods of the Standard American Diet (S.A.D.). This change is sadly reflected in the doubling of diabetes prevalence from 1990 to 2005. Simple carbohydrates, found in highly processed foods such as pastries, breads, cookies, pasta, pizza, and potato chips (just to name a few), tax the body's ability to handle glucose metabolism, which eventually decreases insulin sensitivity. The body's difficulty to handle glucose metabolism occurs because simple carbohydrates (glucose and fructose) cause a spike in blood sugar. The body immediately responds by secreting insulin to lower blood sugar. When a person repeatedly consumes a diet high in simple carbohydrates, it requires a tremendous amount of insulin production, which has the dual effect of decreasing insulin sensitivity, and ultimately, exhausting insulin production and secretion.

HIGH BLOOD PRESSURE AND DEHYDRATION

In regulating water distribution, histamine is produced in response to a water shortage mainly because it stimulates the production of vasopressin, renin, and angiotensin, which (guess what?) causes a rise in blood pressure. Why? Normally, the ratio of water inside the cells (intracellular) to water outside the cells (extracellular) is 1.1:1 (just a little more water is inside the cell than outside). When a water shortage occurs, this ratio changes to 0.8:1 (reverses to more on the outside). In order to get water into the cells, blood pressure must be raised to "inject" water into the cells. Everything our body does is purposeful. It has a reason for raising blood pressure. The body is an amazing adaptive organism. Unfortunately, the medical profession doesn't see it that way.

The renin-angiotensin system is activated by histamine and causes the body to: 1) retain sodium, and consequently, water, 2) stimulate increased water intake (thirst signals), and 3) produce vasoconstriction.

Vasopressin regulates the flow of water into specific cells in the body (higher priority cells such as nerve cells). As Dr. Batmanghelidj aptly describes this situation, "When vasopressin reaches the cell membrane and fuses with its specially designed receptor, the receptor converts to a 'shower head' structure and makes possible filtration of water only through its holes." [4] Vasopressin also causes vasoconstriction of the local capillaries in the area it activates.

The odds are good that most people will have high blood pressure during their lifetimes. In fact, more than 73 million adults have high blood pressure. Approximately 90% of adults with normal blood pressure at age 55 will develop high blood pressure as they get older.

How do conventional medical doctors treat patients with high blood pressure? By giving them water? No. They give them Beta Blockers to lower blood pressure. A Beta Blocker is a medication that slows the heart rate and reduces the force with which the heart muscle contracts, thereby lowering blood pressure. Beta Blockers slow the heart rate by blocking beta-adrenergic receptors in the heart, which prevents adrenaline (epinephrine) from stimulating these receptors. So instead of correcting the problem's cause (dehydration causing high blood pressure) by getting the patient to drink more water, doctors give patients a drug to over-ride the body's natural response to dehydration. Worse yet, sometimes diuretics are prescribed, making a person even more dehydrated! How crazy is that?!

In this chapter, we've seen the ludicrous (especially with high blood pressure) mismanagement of these diseases by modern medicine. That's because modern medicine doesn't seem to care about what's causing disease. For too long, people have believed and trusted medical doctors when most of them are nothing more than technicians. A technician may be able to diagnose a disease, but he thinks nothing of its cause. All he or she does is routinely prescribe the appropriate medication that matches the diagnosis. A true physician looks to the cause of disease. Since our medical system fails to look at causes, you must learn to do it for yourself.

CHAPTER SEVEN

VACCINATION

When you believe in things that you don't understand,
then you suffer. Superstition is a waste.
— **Stevie Wonder**

Stevie Wonder's song "Superstition" is the perfect introduction to the topic of vaccinations. I love his definition of superstition—"when you believe in things that you don't understand." Ninety-nine percent of Americans **do not understand vaccines**, and yet, they believe in them wholeheartedly. Consequently, a great deal of suffering results that no one hears about—largely because no one looks to vaccines as the cause of various health problems. This chapter will give you information about the true nature of vaccines so you can make an educated choice about receiving them.

VACCINATION'S BEGINNINGS

To understand vaccinations, we need to go back to their beginnings.

Thomas Carlyle said, "no error is fully confuted until we have seen not only that it is an error, but how it became one." So let us go back to 1796 to find out how vaccinations began. At the time, bloodletting (using leeches) was still a common practice. It was a very superstitious time "when live frogs were swallowed for the cure of worms; when cow dung and human excreta were mixed with milk and butter for diphtheria; when the brains of a man who had died a violent death were given in teaspoonful doses for the cure of smallpox." [1]

This era was also a very filthy and unsanitary one. Over a century later, Dr. Hadwen would remark of the eighteenth century, "Sanitary arrangements were altogether absent. They obtained their water from conduits and wells in the neighborhood. Water closets (toilets) there were none, and no drainage system existed."

At that time, a man named Edward Jenner decided to seek his fame and fortune. But how would he do it? He wasn't a physician, although he wanted to be one. He couldn't afford the education required so he apprenticed with a surgeon, and then struck out on his own. Although he had never passed a medical examination in his life, Jenner hung up the sign "Surgeon, apothecary" over his door. Not until twenty years after he was in practice did he think it advisable to get a few letters after his name. He then communicated with a Scottish University to obtain the degree of Doctor of Medicine for a mere fifteen pounds. [2]

Jenner had heard the Gloucestershire dairy maids' superstition that if you contract cowpox, then you can't get smallpox. Interested in finding out whether this belief was true, he mentioned it at the local Medico-Convivial Society, where doctors got together to "smoke their pipes, drink their glasses of grog, and talk over their cases." Jenner had no sooner mentioned the superstition than his medical colleagues laughed at it. [3]

Not to be dissuaded, Jenner performed his first experiment on an eight-year old boy named James Phipps. Jenner inoculated Phipps with cowpox and then a short time after with smallpox. When the boy did not contract smallpox, Jenner was elated. "Now," said Jenner, "is the grand discovery. This will answer to my purpose, and I shall soon be able to get another paper for the Royal Society, to follow in the wake of the glorious cuckoo, which has been wittily termed the bird that laid the vaccination egg." [4] Mr. Jenner had previously written an extraordinary paper on the fabulous cuckoo and submitted it to the Royal Society, which his biographer and apologist, Dr. Norman Moore, confessed was how Jenner obtained a Fellowship in the Royal Society. According to Dr. Hadwen, this paper was "for the most part composed of arrant absurdities and imaginative freaks such as no ornithologist of the present day would pay the slightest heed to." [5]

After inoculating James Phipps, Jenner went about the neighborhood aimlessly collecting information regarding cowpox and cowpox milkers. As Sherri Tenpenny points out in her book *Saying No to Vaccines,* "What is not generally discussed about this discovery is that Phipps had been re-vaccinated more than 20 times and died at the age of 20. Jenner also experimented with his own son by inoculation, and his son died at the age of 21. Before their deaths, these boys acquired tuberculosis, which some researchers have linked to the smallpox vaccine." [6]

Jenner then inoculated with smallpox some paupers over 60 years of age, who had contracted the cowpox many years before to see if they would become ill. They did not get smallpox because as people get advanced in life they are more or less immune against it. "This" said Jenner, "is the grand proof of the value of the inoculation of cowpox as a preventive of smallpox." [7] He presented a paper to the Royal Society, taking care never to mention the younger people who had cowpox and yet did get smallpox afterwards. However, the cowpox doctors declared his paper to be rubbish and provided numerous cases as evidence of people who had cowpox only later also to contract smallpox.

Jenner, quickly changing his tune, then came up with the novel idea that there were two kinds of cowpox—the genuine kind, which was never followed by smallpox infection, and the spurious kind in which smallpox did take hold following cowpox inoculation or infection. Next, he sought out the source of the genuine kind. As John Drake describes the situation in *Vaccination Horror*:

> Accordingly, on going into a stable one day he found that a cow had been affected by a very peculiar kind of disease that was produced in this way. It seems that a man had been seeing to the grease upon a horse's heels, and had gone to milk the cows without washing his hands. The result was that it produced that peculiar kind of disease known as horse-grease cowpox. "This," said Jenner "is the life preserving fluid."

It was necessary to perform an experiment, so Jenner inoculated a boy named John Baker with horse-grease. He intended to follow this up by inoculating the boy with smallpox to see if it would take, but instead, the boy died in the workhouse immediately after from having contracted a contagious fever that resulted from the inoculation. [8]

Undeterred, Jenner then inoculated six children with horse-grease cowpox and before waiting to see the results, immediately sent his paper to London to get it printed. Unfortunately for him, as soon as the paper was published, the public outcry was tremendous. As John Drake in *Vaccination Horror*, explains, the result was quite ironic:

> "What," said the people "take horse-grease? Filthy grease from horses' heels, take that and put it into the blood of a child?" No, they would have nothing to do with it. Dr. Pearson wrote Jenner telling him he must take the horse out or "it would damn the whole thing." [9]

Yes, these people denounced horse-grease cowpox, but they were prepared to accept spontaneous cowpox—there's no accounting for taste.

Did Jenner stand and fight for his creed? No, he wanted money, so if the people wanted cowpox, they would get it. Accordingly, he wrote a third paper and tried to wipe out what he had written before. With the exception of a solitary footnote in that paper, horse-grease cowpox was not mentioned at all, and Jenner fell back on the spontaneous cowpox theory he had previously denounced as useless and unprotective.

The twists and turns, the back-pedaling, the lack of concern for the truth and the complete reversal of statements in Jenner's story are remarkable. By distorting the truth and through faulty research, Mr. Jenner, the Father of Vaccines, was raised to legendary status. In return for his efforts the British government paid him enough to make him the equivalent of a multi-millionaire today.

Despite Jenner's efforts, today we now know that cowpox and smallpox are two separate and distinct diseases. You cannot get one from the other, nor can one give immunity to the other. Cowpox is a disease that occurs on the teats of cows. It only occurs in females on the teats and only when they are in milk. According to John Drake the difference is that:

> It [cowpox] results in an ugly chancre and is not infectious. Smallpox, on the other hand, is not limited to the female sex as is cow-pox, nor to one portion of the body; it presents different physical signs, and, furthermore, is tremendously infectious, and the course and symptoms of the two diseases are totally different. [10]

THE STATISTICS OF THE TIMES

What resulted from these vaccinations? Parliament passed the Act of 1853, which mandated that everyone get vaccinated or pay a fine. Sherri Tenpenny points out that, "Since the passing of the Act in 1853 we have had no less than three distinct epidemics. In 1857-9 we had more than 14,000 deaths from smallpox; in the 1863-5 epidemic the deaths had increased to 20,000; and in 1871-2 they totaled up to 44,800." [11] The population did increase by 7 percent, but the smallpox deaths increased by 41 percent. Between the second and third epidemics, the population increased by 9 percent and the smallpox by 120 percent! It surely appears that rather than prevent an epidemic, vaccinations created them.

In a report published in an early edition of *The British Medical Journal*, Dr. L. Parry asked the following questions regarding nineteenth century vaccination statistics:

> How is it that smallpox is five times as likely to be fatal in the vaccinated as the unvaccinated? How is it that in some of our highest vaccinated towns—for example, Bombay and Calcutta—smallpox is rife, whilst in some of our most poorly vaccinated towns, such as Leicester, it is almost unknown? How is it that almost 80 percent have been vaccinated, whilst only 20 percent have not been vaccinated?

Note that just prior to Dr. Parry's comments, Leicester had experienced a smallpox epidemic following a mandatory vaccination until the people rebelled against the vaccination. [12]

Through the last two centuries and across the globe, mandatory vaccinations always coincided with smallpox and other epidemics. When the people finally revolted against mandatory vaccinations, they were terminated, and not surprisingly, the epidemics also sharply declined. This situation has repeated itself all over the world in the 1800s and 1900s. Statistics showing the absolute correlation between vaccination and disease are abundant. For the purpose of brevity, I will include just a few of the many crystal clear statistics.

For a period of time, Mexico, with its rigidly enforced vaccination laws, had the world's worst record of smallpox deaths. The following chart shows the comparison between Mexico with its sparse population of 16,500,000 (circa 1930) and British India with its dense, congested population (300,000,000 approximately). In spite of the disease breeding conditions of India's cities with inadequate sanitation, nutrition, and housing facilities and the polluted water, lack of sewers, and extreme heat, the smallpox death rate was far lower than that of completely vaccinated Mexico.

SMALLPOX DEATHS AND DEATH RATES PER MILLION PEOPLE				
	MEXICO		BRITISH/INDIA	
Year	Deaths	Death Rate	Deaths	Death Rate
1922	11,966	844	40,836	169
1923	13,074	903	44,084	183
1924	11,964	878	55,380	229
1925	11,003	731	86,986	356
1926	5,477	357	117,086	485
1927	6,639	424	118,197	490
1928	6,694	420	96,133	399
1929	11,304	696	72,884	302
1930	17,405	1,053	71,815	140
1931	14,903	886	37,272	167
1932	8,307	485	44,925	183

Other diseases also showed a strong correlation between vaccination and rate of illness and death. [13]

CHART SHOWING INCREASE IN DISEASE BEFORE AND AFTER VACCINATION CAMPAIGN [14]		
DISEASES	APRIL 3, 1954	JULY 10, 1954
(Annually to date)	Before Vaccinations	After Vacc. Campaign
Chickenpox	6,684	13,515
Measles (also German)	4,056	13,912
Mumps	2,182	5,196
Scarlet fever	1,256	2,295
Syphilis	828	1,631
Total of the 48 diseases recorded	19,997	47,070

CANCER AND OTHER DISEASES CAUSED BY VACCINATION

Many doctors, after years of experience with vaccinations, have come to the sober conclusion that vaccinations not only do not prevent disease, but in fact cause many diseases.

Dr. Alexander Wilder, editor of the *New York Medical Times*, Professor of Pathology in the United States Medical College of New York and author of *Wilder's History of Medicine*, made this observation:

Vaccination is the infusion of [a] contaminating element into the system, and after such contamination you can never be sure of regaining the former purity of the body. Consumption follows in the wake of vaccination as surely as effect follows cause. [15]

Dr. Walter M. James of Philadelphia says:

> Vaccination does not stay the spread of smallpox nor even modify it in those who get it after vaccination. It does introduce into the system, and therefore contributes to the spread of tuberculosis, cancer and even leprosy. It tends to make more virulent epidemics of smallpox and to make them more extensive. It does just what inoculation did—cause the spread of disease. [16]

You might be thinking to yourself, "How can this be? What mechanism could be at work, causing this to happen?" The answer is one of the great paradoxes—one could even say hypocrisies—of modern medicine. On the one hand, hospitals and surgeons in particular are incredibly conscientious about aseptic surgery and cleanliness. They wash their hands and don rubber gloves and face-masks for surgery. Everything is carefully sterilized before and after surgery. People are even told to wash their hands before eating and after using the restroom, or especially after coming in contact with a sick person.

And then they go and stick a needle filled with filthy, infectious poison directly into the bloodstream. *Am I the only one astounded by this logic?* (Actually I know I'm not, thank God.)

The medical establishment reasons that by introducing the diseased element into the bloodstream, it will stimulate the body's production of antibodies to fight off the "potential" invader, thereby strengthening immunity. But I beg to differ.

LEVELS OF DEFENSE

Imagine a castle under siege. Every well-built castle has levels of defense. Usually a great open field surrounds all sides of the castle so invaders can be seen coming "a mile away." Often a moat (water obstacle) also surrounds the castle, with a single bridge or draw-bridge. The next obstacle is the outer castle wall, lined with soldiers and archers, perhaps even cannons. If the outer wall is breached, the soldiers retreat to a deeper level of the fortress. But what if the enemy knew of a secret underground passage into the castle's heart? What if, while the soldiers are busy patrolling the outer walls, the enemy sprang from within the heart of the castle? I daresay the odds don't look too good for the defenders. One can easily imagine the chaos, confusion, and frustration of the defending army. The soldiers are wondering, "Where did they (the enemy) come from?" Actually, the soldiers might be killed before they even have time to contemplate the question.

This is exactly the situation your body faces when a filthy foreign element is introduced directly into your bloodstream (vaccination). It's like your enemies coming in the back door, where you least expect them to enter; only someone opened the door and escorted them in.

Your body also has levels of defense. Your skin provides an effective barrier to foreign substances and potential invaders. Outside of a cut (a breach in the outer wall), *normally* only two ways exist for a foreign invader to get in: 1) your nose and respiratory tract, or 2) your mouth and digestive tract. Both the respiratory and digestive tracts are lined with front-line defenders of the immune system. When an invader is detected, the immune system mobilizes more of its army. A common cold or even flu is your body's natural defense to throwing off toxins or an infectious agent.

Actually, an infection can only take hold when your body has become a toxic breeding ground for disease. As we learned in a previous chapter, a toxic environment is an acidic one, ripe for disease to flourish. Bacteria and viruses require an acidic, oxygen-deficient environment to survive and thrive. An infection is really the body's way of throwing off the poisons that have accumulated. Just as worms and bacteria decompose waste products, the bacteria and viruses in your body also actually help to break down waste, so your body can get rid of it. Normally, "bad bacteria" is already present in your digestive tract, but kept in check by a healthy, clean, alkaline environment. When you take antibiotics, you suppress this cleansing function of the body, thereby allowing waste products and toxins to build up, setting the stage for chronic degenerative diseases.

The bacteria and viruses are still only as deep into your body's fortress as the digestive and/or respiratory tract. They still have not penetrated into the bloodstream. Your body is made this way for a reason; your blood delivers oxygen and nutrients to all your body's cells and takes carbon dioxide and other waste products away to be eliminated from the body because your body is meant to be pure and clean. Consider gangrene. Doctors know that a gangrenous wound (an infection which is about to penetrate into the bloodstream) needs to be surgically removed (even if it means the loss of a limb) or the patient will die of blood poisoning.

Just as the army defending the castle was bewildered and frustrated by the enemy that found a secret passage into the castle's heart, your poor body can be overwhelmed by the poisonous vaccine introduced directly into the bloodstream. Imagine how you would react if you were part of that bewildered army. With every insult (vaccination), your immune system grows weaker and more dysfunctional. It grows weaker because it's constantly on the defensive; once an infectious or foreign agent makes it into the bloodstream, it is very difficult for your body to get rid of it. Your body grows more dysfunctional because it doesn't know who or where the enemy is anymore. So it starts attacking its own kind. I believe this attack is the root of many if not most autoimmune diseases, and I'm not alone in this belief.

You may recall from the heart disease chapter that when a microbial invasion occurs, the immune system produces free radical scavengers to help destroy the microbial invaders. But that process includes a lot of "friendly fire," which causes cellular destruction and inflammation, now known as a major cause of atherosclerosis, and thus heart disease. When an infectious agent is introduced into the bloodstream, as in vaccination, the immune system is on constant alert; once the infectious agent is in the bloodstream, it is very difficult for the body to eliminate it completely and it becomes an ongoing threat. The body is continually mobilizing the immune system's warriors, and inflammation, thought by many to be the cause of most diseases, is continually produced in the body. No wonder researchers have said that vaccinations also increase the rate of heart disease.

Dr. J. W. Hodge had considerable experience with vaccination before he denounced it and wrote a book on his collected data. In his book *The Vaccination Superstition*, he states:

After a thorough investigation of the most authentic records and facts in harmony with the physician's daily observations and experiences, the conclusion is drawn that instead of protecting its subjects from contagion of smallpox, vaccination actually renders them more susceptible to it. *Vaccination is the implantation of disease*—that is its admitted purpose. Health is the ideal state to be sought, not disease…Every pathogenic disturbance in the infected organism wastes and lowers the vital powers, and thus diminishes its natural resisting capacity. [17]

VACCINES AND YOUR IMMUNE SYSTEM

What effect do vaccines have on your immune system? Vaccines are deemed effective if they produce antibodies. One incorrect assumption about vaccines is that "effectiveness" and "protectiveness" are the same thing. Studies have repeatedly shown that the production of antibodies has not proven to correlate with protection. So what does confer lifetime immunity? Your immune system is capable of remembering a virus you had, such as measles or chicken pox, and then knows immediately to eliminate that virus when it tries to reenter without your having to experience the infection again. [18]

Your immune system functions in two ways: 1) Humoral (in the bloodstream) involves the production of antibodies, and 2) Cell-mediated includes different types of white blood cells, including macrophages and several different lymphocytes. This teamwork between the humoral and cell-mediated divisions records the infection as a long-term memory to provide immunity, like a lifelong insurance protection policy against ever contracting the infection again. [19]

In other words, because vaccines stimulate only antibody production in the bloodstream, they do not involve the cell-mediated division, which is necessary to confer the long-term memory. This long-term memory provides the lifetime protection. Why would vaccines stimulate only antibody production in the bloodstream and not in the cell-mediated division? Because the foreign invaders are ONLY in the bloodstream (thanks to the vaccine).

In an infant, "lymphocytes can differentiate into either TH1 cells, representing a predominance of cell mediated immunity, or TH2 cells, a preponderance of humeral antibody immunity. A healthy immune system has a bias toward the TH1 system" (cell-mediated). [20] Vaccines, however, shift the immune system heavily toward TH2 (humoral antibody) dominance. As Sherri Tenpenny explains,

"Persons with a TH2-skewed immune response tend to have allergies and asthma. The increased TH2 pattern has also been associated with increases in autoimmune disorders, type 1 diabetes, inflammatory bowel disease and autism." [21]

ADDITIVES

More than 100 different additives, chemicals, preservatives, and antibiotics are added to different vaccines, with each vaccine containing considerable amounts of most of these, and trace amounts of others. Included are formaldehyde, aluminum hydroxide, mercury (thimerosal), antibiotics such as streptomycin and neomycin, gelatin, phenoxyethanol (anti-freeze), monosodium glutamate (MSG), and polysorbate 80. Formaldehyde, a preservative, is a known carcinogen. Aluminum hydroxide is used as an adjuvant to stimulate an immune response; it induces the production of IgE antibodies, "the antibody present in most persons with allergies." [22] Another adjuvant now coming into use is squalene. It is naturally manufactured in the liver and is also contained in shark liver oil, so it appears to be a good choice. "However, ingested squalene has a completely different effect on the body than injected squalene. When molecules of squalene enter the body through an injection, even at concentrations as small as 10 to 20 parts per billion, it can lead to self-destructive immune responses, such as autoimmune arthritis and lupus." [23] Mercury, or thimerosal, "can induce a strong increase of IgE. Mercury depletes glutathione, polarizing the TH2 dominance." [24] Gelatin also causes a strong rise in IgE levels, and is known to have caused anaphylaxis in many children. "Anaphylaxis to gelatin is the most common identifiable cause of severe allergic reaction to vaccine." [25]

The use of all these additives in vaccines for children has been challenged by Jack Doubleday, CEO of the California non-profit, Natural Woman, Natural Man, Inc. In January of 2001, he "offered $20,000 to the first U.S.-licensed medical doctor or pharmaceutical company CEO who would publicly drink a standard mixture of vaccine additive ingredients. On August 1, 2007, the offer was increased to $90,000 and will increase $5,000 per month, in perpetuity, until a medical doctor, a pharmaceutical executive, or any of the 15 current members of the ACIP agrees to drink a dose of chemicals that would be the dose given to an infant." [26] All I can say is "Wow!"

At the time of this writing (early 2010), the pot offered by Jack Doubleday has increased to nearly a quarter of a million dollars. If a person were to start medical school now, by the time he or she graduates (four years hence), the pot will be nearly half a million dollars. The cost and grind of medical school and the toxic effect of these additives may just be worth enduring.

Many vaccines also contain stray viruses and bacterial contamination. These viruses and bacteria have been known to result in illness in many people as well as mortality in others.

123

SERIOUS ADVERSE REACTIONS

Every year, the Vaccine Adverse Event Reporting System (VAERS) has an estimated 11,000 to 12,000 reports of vaccine reactions filed with it. According to the *Journal of the American Medical Association* (*JAMA*):

> Between mid-1999 and January 4, 2004, a total of 128,035 adverse reactions were reported to VAERS. Because it is estimated that only 1 percent of all adverse drug reactions are voluntarily reported, this figure may actually represent 1.28 million adverse reactions. During that same period, 2,093 deaths occurred soon after vaccinations were reported to VAERS. This may actually represent between 20,930 (1 percent) and 209,300 (10 percent) of all deaths possibly associated with vaccines. [27]

A Vaccine Court, with appointed judges, hears the cases of those injured by vaccines. "Even though more than $1 billion has been paid to vaccine-injured victims, only 20 percent of persons who apply receive compensation." [28] This fact indicates that if 100% were heard in court, $5 billion would have been paid out in compensation!

FEAR TACTICS

Parents (and adults in general), doctors, public health officials, the pharmaceutical industry, and the media all constantly drill into us the fear that there will be adverse consequences if we do NOT get vaccinated. Recently, radio and television stations were bemoaning the lack of available swine flu vaccines as if it were the world's greatest tragedy. A 1963 guide published by the Federal Communicable Disease Center (former name for the CDC) contended that, "the full use of the word epidemic in public statements is the most effective single means of stimulating the public to action." [29]

THE FINANCIAL PAYOFF

In *Saying No to Vaccines*, Dr. Tenpenny takes on the aggressive behavior of pharmaceutical companies in their promotion for vaccinations:

Today the clout of the immense pharmaceutical giants is used to persuade and coerce state and national government officials to embrace massive, expensive vaccination programs. For example, over the last seven years, the industry has contributed more than $800 million in federal and state lobbying and campaign donations. No other industry has spent more money to sway public policy to use their products: drugs and vaccines. [30]

While the pharmaceutical industry is spending more than $100 million a year to coerce and persuade government officials to embrace its massive, expensive vaccination programs, it's certainly no vain effort.

In 1900 the only vaccine given to school children was smallpox; by 1971 smallpox had been eradicated and the vaccine was no longer required for school. As recently as 1985, the only vaccines required for school were polio, diphtheria-tetanus-pertussis

(DTP) and measles-mumps-rubella (MMR). By 2007, 113 vaccine antigens from at least 10 different vaccines had been added as school requirements. [31]

Charles Hoppe, a Brooklyn theosophist, said in 1931, "It is revolting, to say the least, to think I must have diseased animal matter injected into the blood of my child before he can receive an education." [32]

Vaccines are costing the country billions in tax dollars and healthcare costs. In 2005, "The global vaccine market is generating between $10 billion and $16 billion dollars per year. The global vaccine business is projected to grow 18 percent a year to $30 billion by 2011, well above the 4.4 percent annual growth expected for the drug industry overall." [33] No wonder healthcare costs are astronomical!

Vaccines not only produce direct revenue, but they also increase the use of drugs to treat all of the disease conditions resulting from vaccinations. It's difficult to imagine all of the diseases that have been caused by vaccinations and the costs of treating them.

If you are not yet convinced of the devastatingly detrimental effects of vaccines, I strongly encourage you to read Eleanor McBean's book, *The Poisoned Needle*. Another excellent book is Dr. Sherri Tenpenny's *Saying No to Vaccines*. In her book, Dr. Tenpenny also includes "vaccine exemptions for schools, healthcare, military and other special circumstances." This is an incredibly well researched and highly informative book that is also highly readable.

When I set out to write this book, this chapter was sort of an afterthought, the last I wrote, but now it has become my favorite chapter. Why? Because to me, vaccinations represent the epitome of medical ignorance, as well as the ruthless greed of pharmaceutical companies. I think the discussion here has demonstrated that pretty clearly. I hope it has armed the reader with enough knowledge and self-assurance confidently to "Just Say NO to Vaccines."

PART TWO

A BLUEPRINT FOR RADIANT
HEALTH AND WELLNESS

In Part One, the reader hopefully cleared the hurdle of Big Medicine's programming. The importance of adequate water consumption—which is the single most important and yet overlooked aspect of health—should also be crystal clear. The value of ionized, hexagonal water is inestimable—I believe that buying a water ionizer for the home (and using it daily) is the best investment a person can make for his or her health.

In Part Two, we're going to shift gears to look at what I feel to be the most important factors related to health. Consider for a moment a master gardener. He (or she) is so conscientious about making sure his vegetable or flower garden has all the proper nutrients and conditions favorable to the plant. He faithfully gives it sufficient water on a regular basis, and often, he will moderate the amount of sun the plants receive with shading. If a cold snap is on the way, he will spray the leaves with a sugary (molasses) nutrient-rich mixture to strengthen it. If the plant or tree becomes sick, or infested with some bacteria, virus, mold or other microorganism, he will make every effort to find out the cause and its remedy. For their efforts, master gardeners are rewarded with a bountiful harvest or beautiful blooms they may enjoy!

If people gave as much care to their bodies as a master gardener does to his plants, then everyone would be much healthier. But very few people provide themselves with adequate care. This situation has always been a mystery to me. If master gardeners know everything needed for the healthy growth of their plants and trees, and even how to care for them in disease, why aren't we able to do the same for own our bodies? For some reason, people think, "If the medical doctors can't figure out how to cure me, there's no way I can." People are so lazy they don't even make much of an effort to learn what nutrients and conditions their bodies need to be healthy. They take a very passive role in their own health and healthcare, and then act like they can't believe it when they get sick—as though it's just bad luck! They feel victimized by their own bodies, which they are each ultimately responsible for as the body's leader.

If the reader will garner understanding of how to care for his or her body, and care for its well-being like a master gardener cares for his garden, the reader will most certainly reap the rewards as well.

CHAPTER EIGHT

DIET AND NUTRITION

Let food be your medicine.

— **Hippocrates**

WHOLE FOODS VS. PROCESSED FOODS

This chapter's purpose is to demonstrate that the more whole foods your diet contains, and the less processed foods you eat, the healthier you will become. It's really that simple. In this chapter, I will give repeated examples showing the vast difference between the effects of whole foods and processed foods in your body. The Standard American Diet (S.A.D.) is sadly very high in processed foods, and very low in whole foods. How can a state of health possibly result from consuming such a diet? What would happen to your car if you filled it with sugar water instead of gasoline? If people even cared for their bodies like they care for their cars, we would be much healthier as a nation. Most processed foods have almost no nutritive value (actually most processed foods take more nutrients out of your body than they provide) while at the same time, they contain an abundance of toxic chemicals and other health-degrading substances.

In order fully to understand healthy nutrition, we need to have a basic understanding of the nutrients that our body requires, and some of the roles these vital nutrients play in our bodies. It's also important to keep in mind that these nutrients work together, in terms of absorption and assimilation into the body. Additionally, a proper balance is necessary between them for the body to use them properly. As an example, calcium absorption requires the presence of magnesium in the diet at a certain ratio, once thought to be 2:1 (calcium to magnesium). Many researchers are now advocating a 1:1 ratio, while some are even suggesting a 2:1 ratio of magnesium to calcium. This 2:1 ratio corresponds more closely to the ratio naturally found in a grain-and-vegetable-based diet. In fact, a balanced whole food diet contains a favorable mix of all known nutrients essential for calcium absorption. [1]

As mentioned earlier, for calcium to be effectively incorporated into the skeletal structure, at least 50% of the dietary fats should be saturated. Additionally, Vitamin D, a vital fat-soluble vitamin, is needed for many vital body parts and functions involving calcium, including healthy bones and a healthy nervous system, proper growth, mineral metabolism, and muscle tone. Cholesterol is a precursor to Vitamin D.

Chlorophyll, a product of photosynthesis, is vitally important as a regulator of calcium. When sunlight touches plants, it produces chlorophyll, most abundantly in green plants. Chlorophyll and hemoglobin (a major component of red blood cells) are structurally identical, except that at the center of the hemoglobin molecule is iron. In chlorophyll, that element is magnesium. Foods containing chlorophyll act like stored sunshine (Vitamin D) by regulating calcium metabolism. In addition, most green plants, because they contain sources of phosphorous and Vitamins A and C, also are important for calcium absorption.

As this information shows, all nutrients have an interconnectedness; for this reason, a whole foods diet is essential to optimal nutrition and health.

PROTEINS

Your body assembles and utilizes some 50,000 different proteins to build and repair all its tissues. Every cell in every organ is built from these different proteins, giving them a unique structure and function. Enzymes that catalyze chemical processes, antibodies of the immune system, and most hormones are specialized proteins. Amino acids, the building blocks of proteins, are involved in most of the body's processes and functions. In other words, proteins and the amino acids that comprise them all have specific body functions. There are 22 amino acids that combine together to make the different proteins in your body, eight of which are essential amino acids because the body cannot manufacture them on its own.

Through the years, much debate has been waged over the healthiness of vegetarianism vs. a diet containing animal protein. Vegetarians claim that all the body's required amino acids and proteins can be found in a plant-based diet while a diet containing meat can lead to cancer. Meat eaters say that animal protein is our only source of complete protein. Vegetarians admit that in order to provide all the essential amino acids, they need to consume grains and legumes (beans, peas, and lentils) together.

In the vegetable kingdom, the two best sources of protein are legumes (beans) and cereal grains—amino acids that may be lacking in one are filled by the other, and vice versa. Therefore, to get the best amino acid combination, beans and grains should be eaten together, preferably with at least a small amount of (animal) protein.

Additionally, usable Vitamin B_{12} occurs only in animal products. According to the authors of *Nourishing Traditions,* "The B_{12} contained in fermented soy products and micro-algae such as spirulina are not absorbed by humans because they are not picked up by the 'intrinsic factor' a specialized protein secreted by the stomach that allows B_{12} to be assimilated." [2]

Research studies that link meat eating with cancer, in particular of the colon, do not take into account that these diets often also contain high levels of omega-6 linoleic acid and hydrogenated fats, which in themselves are known cancer-causing agents.

Meat is also rich in many important minerals such as phosphorous, iron, and zinc. A vegetarian diet also lacks the fat-soluble catalysts for mineral absorption. Fallon and Egan argue that, "In humans, zinc deficiency can cause learning disabilities and mental retardation. In men, zinc depletion reduces fertility. Men's best source of zinc is animal products, particularly oysters and red meat." [3]

Animal products supply a wealth of complete proteins, fats, minerals, and Vitamins B_6 and B_{12}. In their whole form, these all work together to aid in assimilation in the body. One problem with today's diet is that fats, especially saturated animal fats, have been labeled the bad guy. Consequently, much or all of the fat has been removed from milk.

Fallon and Egan note about animal protein foods, "We cannot stress too highly that animal protein foods—meat, eggs, and milk—always come with fat and this is how we should eat them." Americans, however, routinely buy low- or non-fat milk, go for the leanest ground beef, and take the skin off the chicken, thinking it's the healthy thing to do. It's not. "Animal fat supplies vitamins A and D needed for the assimilation of protein. Consumption of low-fat milk products, egg whites and lean meat can lead to serious deficiencies of these vital fat-soluble nutrients." [4]

Finally, a major concern with most of the animal products available in the supermarkets is the way the animals have been raised. Most cattle, pigs, and chickens are raised in very confined spaces and grain-fed, which presents a number of problems. Because of the confined living spaces, disease is rampant, so antibiotics are given routinely. However, diseased animals still find their way into the food supply. Calves raised for veal are confined to crates for the whole of their short pathetic lives. Steroids and growth hormones are given to speed up growth and tenderize the meat. Instead of "free-ranging," chickens are confined to crowded pens, often under artificial light night and day (to increase egg production) and fed on substandard food. The cramped quarters and lack of exercise makes for very unhealthy and neurotic chickens. The sad result is that they often end up pecking each other to death. Without their normal diet of grass and insects, these chickens provide meat and eggs that are sorely lacking in nutritional value. Beef from cattle and milk from cows are also less nutritious on a grain-fed diet, compared to one mostly consisting of grass. For moral as well as health concerns, organic and free-range chickens and beef are the best choice.

OILS AND FATS: WHOLE VS. PROCESSED

You may recall that over a sixty year period, where traditional animal fat in the American diet declined and butter consumption plummeted, the percentage of dietary vegetable oils in the form of margarine, shortening, and refined oils increased about 400%. At the same time, deaths due to heart disease skyrocketed. Let's take a closer look at why.

Butter and traditional animal fats are naturally saturated, which means that all available spaces for hydrogen atoms are filled, making for a very stable fat or oil. Fats and oils are vulnerable to rancidity or oxidation, which turns them into trans fats or free radicals. Saturated fats, being more stable, are less likely to become oxidized or turn rancid. For this reason, the food industry hydrogenates oils (adds hydrogen atoms) to turn them into more stable saturated fats, such as margarine or shortening. This extends shelf life, thereby saving the food industry a lot of money, which increases profits.

Let's take a closer look at the processing of oils and fats, starting with extraction.

Oils from fruits, nuts, and seeds first need to be extracted. In the old days, slow-moving stone presses did this work, but in today's high-tech world, speed equals money. So the oil is processed in large factories first by crushing the oil-bearing seeds and nuts and heating them to 230 degrees Fahrenheit. During this process, the oil is further damaged by exposure to light and oxygen. The oil is then squeezed out at high pressures (10 to 20 tons per inch), generating even more heat. Toxic solvents, such as hexane, are added to extract the last bit of oil. Chemical preservatives such as BHT and BHA are added to replace the Vitamin E and other natural preservatives destroyed in the high heat.

Fallon and Enig explain:

> One reason the polyunsaturates cause so many health problems is that they tend to become oxidized or rancid when subjected to heat, oxygen and moisture as in cooking and processing. Rancid oils are characterized by free radicals—that is, single atoms or clusters with an unpaired electron in an outer orbit. [5]

Most of the commonly used "vegetable" oils, such as canola, soy, corn, safflower, sunflower, peanut, and sesame are polyunsaturated oils. Since these oils are less stable, by the time polyunsaturated oils are done being processed, they are very likely already free radicals. Fallon and Enig conclude, "These compounds are extremely reactive chemically. They have been characterized as 'marauders' in the body for they attack cell membranes and red blood cells, causing damage in DNA/RNA strands that can trigger mutations in tissue, blood vessels and skin." [6]

Hydrogenation is the next insult. Its main purpose is to increase shelf life by turning oils into fats that are solid at room temperature—margarine and shortening. This process takes the cheapest polyunsaturated oils—soy, corn, canola, or cottonseed, already rancid from the extraction process—and subjects them to further high pressure and high temperature. A catalyst, usually nickel oxide, is added prior to the high pressure, high heat process. This catalyst causes the hydrogen atoms to change positions on the molecule, changing them from a healthy cis formation (found in nature) to a destructive trans fat. Soap-like emulsifiers are added to give margarine a better consistency. Then the oil is steam-cleaned at high temperatures again to remove unpleasant odors. It is then bleached to remove margarine's natural unappetizing grey color. Dyes and strong flavors are added to make it look and taste like butter.

Although these man-made trans fats are foreign and toxic to the body, unfortunately, your body does not recognize them as such. Instead of being eliminated, these trans fats are incorporated into the cell membranes as though they were cis fats, causing your cells actually to become partially hydrogenated! These trans fats, now part of the cell membranes, wreak havoc with cell metabolism—since electrons in the cell membranes must be in certain arrangements or patterns for chemical reactions to take place. The hydrogenation process disturbs this electron alignment. Margarine, due to its abundance of free radicals, causes chronic high levels of cholesterol and has been linked to both heart disease and cancer because it is loaded with trans fats and free radicals, which cause cellular damage and inflammation. The free radicals damage cellular DNA, directly linked to cancer. Trans fats are also known carcinogens. [7]

It's a miracle of modern marketing that margarine and shortening are considered to be heart healthy fats. When are we going to realize that natural whole foods are what the body wants and needs, not processed fake food?

Butter on the other hand, is actually one of the healthiest and most nourishing foods you can eat (contrary to popular belief). It is rich in the fat-soluble vitamins, which include true Vitamin A or retinol, Vitamin D, Vitamin K, and Vitamin E plus their naturally occurring cofactors that give them their greatest benefit. As Fallon and Egan agree, "Butter is America's best source of these important nutrients." [8]

Butter, being naturally saturated, does not go rancid or get oxidized very easily. It ensures proper assimilation of the minerals and water-soluble vitamins in vegetables, grains, and meat, as well as the protein in meat. Butter has very little lactose, making it readily digestible by almost everyone.

For cooking at moderate to higher temperatures, coconut oil is perhaps the best. Because it is a saturated fat, it holds up well under higher heat, even better than butter.

FAST FOODS

For those who routinely eat at fast food "restaurants," here's a wakeup call from a recent *Natural News* article written by Mike Adams. His article, titled, "Window Cleaning Chemical Injected Into Fast Food Hamburger Meat" is based on another article that appeared in the *New York Times*, so you can be sure everything is as he reports it. I preface it because the truth is sometimes almost ridiculous, as in this case. Here are just a few brief excerpts:

> If you're in the beef business, what do you do with all the extra cow parts and trimmings that have traditionally been sold off for use in pet food? You scrape them together into a pink mass, inject them with a chemical to kill the e. coli, and sell them to fast food restaurants to make into hamburgers.

This process is exactly what McDonald's, Burger King, and most other fast food restaurants have done. What's even more disturbing is that our federal school lunch programs are doing the same thing. The chemical injected to kill bacteria is ammonia, commonly used in glass cleaning and window cleaning products.

> This ammonia-injected beef comes from a company called *Beef Products, Inc.* As *NYT* reports, the federal school lunch program used a whopping 5.5 million pounds of ammonia-injected beef trimmings from this company in 2008.

Perhaps most disturbing of all is the USDA's complicity. "This is all fine with the USDA, which endorses the procedure as a way to make the hamburger beef 'safe' enough to eat. Ammonia kills e. coli, you see, and the USDA doesn't seem to be concerned with the fact that **people are eating ammonia in their hamburgers.**" Furthermore, the USDA agreed to the request of Beef Products Inc. to classify the ammonia as a processing agent, so it need not be listed as an ingredient on labels.

Another problem is that "the ammonia doesn't always kill the pathogens. Both e. coli and salmonella have been found contaminating the cow-derived products sold by this company." [http://www.naturalnews.com/027872_ammonia_beef_products.html]

So let's briefly review. When you order a burger at a fast food joint (restaurant sounds too dignified), you're getting "dog-food-grade" hamburger meat injected with window cleaner, possibly still contaminated with e. coli or salmonella, and the USDA thinks that's just fine! If that doesn't make you want to cook and eat at home more, nothing will.

SALAD DRESSINGS

Most bottled salad dressings are not recommended because they are made with polyunsaturated oils, along with preservatives, artificial flavors, coloring, and refined sweeteners.

The high percentage of oleic acid makes olive oil ideal for salads and for cooking at moderate temperatures. Extra virgin olive oil is also rich in antioxidants. Olive oil has withstood the test of time; it is the safest vegetable oil you can use, but don't overdo it.

Extra virgin olive oil, rather than being processed at high temperatures and high pressures, is produced by crushing olives between stone or steel rollers with minimal exposure to light and oxygen. When used along with raw vinegar or lemon juice, virgin olive oil makes for a healthful and tasty dressing to salads. *Nourishing Traditions* has delicious salad dressing recipes using olive oil and other healthful ingredients. A good basic recipe is 2 parts olive oil to 1 part balsamic or apple cider vinegar, some sea salt, pepper, and some garlic pressed in (unless you plan on kissing someone soon).

CARBOHYDRATES—UNREFINED PLANT FOODS VS. REFINED CARBOHYDRATES

A lot of confusion and debate surrounds carbohydrates. Many "experts" advocate a low or no carbohydrate diet, but I believe the support for such diets is misguided. Low or no carbohydrate diets may work in terms of weight loss, but are they really healthy for the body? Just as we saw how a restricted fat diet can lead to serious deficiencies, the same can occur with carbohydrates. Carbohydrates are necessary for the production of fast, available energy. Among their many vital roles, fats are a good source of slower time-release energy, and also for long-term storage of energy. Unrefined plant foods in the form of whole grains, legumes, vegetables, and fruits also contain a rich supply of vitamins, minerals, and co-factors necessary for your body's optimal functioning.

Why do carbohydrates get a bad rap? Because most (or all) of the ills caused by their consumption come from the consumption of **refined** carbohydrates. What's the difference? One main difference is that refined carbohydrates have been broken down to simple carbohydrates. In whole food form, most carbohydrates are complex. Your body processes simple and complex carbohydrates in different ways. Complex carbohydrates are usually first stored in the liver as glycogen and broken down into glucose when needed. Simple carbohydrates are rapidly digested and released into your blood stream. This flood of simple sugars elevates your blood glucose levels rapidly. Insulin is then produced in abundance by the pancreas to shuttle the glucose into the cells. This big influx of insulin then causes the blood sugar levels to crash. A person then ravenously consumes more simple sugars to elevate blood sugar levels, and the whole vicious cycle repeats itself. The problem is that after a while, insulin sensitivity (of the cell receptors) decreases, or the pancreas may lose its ability to produce sufficient insulin. The result is the modern degenerative disease called type 2 diabetes. The reason diabetes and obesity seem to go hand in hand is probably because all of these simple sugars are then stored in the body as fat.

Another major problem with refined carbohydrates, like most refined and processed foods, is that most of the nutrients have been "processed out" of them or destroyed in the high heat. Meanwhile, all kinds of chemical preservatives, flavorings, colorings, and refined sweeteners have been processed in. Processed foods abound with chemical toxins and free radicals, while being severely depleted of most nutrients.

Paul Pitchford, in his excellent book, *Healing With Whole Foods*, says, "many people are highly deficient in minerals as a result of our food production and processing methods. As such, these deficiencies can lead to degenerative diseases." [9]

Let's take a look at two of the most commonly consumed whole grains: whole wheat and brown rice. These grains, in their whole food form, are incredibly nutrient-rich; while in the processed form (white flour and white rice) commonly consumed by most Americans, they are very poor in nutrients. In fact, almost all of their nutritive value is gone.

Whole wheat is virtually unknown to the average person in its true form. Before it's milled into flour, it's in the form of wheat berries or seeds. These whole-wheat seeds can comprise dozens of minerals and micro-minerals if grown in rich soil. They can also contain immune-protective phytonutrients as well as vitamins and precious oils. In refining, the majority of these nutrients are lost.

Two of these minerals that are lost in processing are selenium and magnesium. Selenium (found abundantly in whole wheat) deficiency can cause low thyroid function or hypothyroid. Normally when one thinks of low thyroid, iodine deficiency first comes to mind. Here we see a little known mineral having a vital function. Obesity and low thyroid are directly related because thyroid function regulates the metabolic rate. Selenium is involved in the transformation of thyroxin (T_4) into triiodothyronine (T_3), which allows for the metabolism of nutrients. Selenium also has the ability to neutralize toxic heavy metals such as lead and mercury by binding with them. [10]

As for magnesium, approximately 70% of the United States population suffers magnesium deficiency, which is considered one of the most under-diagnosed deficiencies. Magnesium has many healing properties. It calms nerve function and causes muscle relaxation. People with frequent muscle spasms and cramps can benefit from including more magnesium-rich foods in their diets. Magnesium also has a calming and harmonizing effect on mental function and the emotions. Its relaxing effect on muscles includes the heart as well as menstrual cramps in PMS (premenstrual syndrome) and migraine headaches. It creates "better digestive flow, relieving constipation; and stabilizes blood sugar imbalances in alcoholism and diabetes." [11]

As we saw earlier in this chapter, magnesium is vitally important in calcium metabolism. It can prevent osteoporosis by pushing calcium into the bones, thereby also averting calcium excesses in the soft tissues, and counteracting conditions such as chronic fatigue syndrome, fibromyalgia, and arthritis.

All this information about calcium leads Pitchford to conclude:

Massive calcium intake without adequate dietary magnesium can lead to another sinister event: calcium tends to deposit in the soft tissues rather than entering the skeleton. Thus, soft-tissue calcium excess, a problem that has been avidly researched for the last thirty years, may predispose one to any degeneration, particularly those of the kidneys, skeleton, heart, and vascular system. [12]

Magnesium also plays a major part in preventing coronary artery disease, as it relaxes smooth muscles (such as those found in the heart), dilates coronary and peripheral blood vessels, helps to prevent blood clotting, and prevents irregular heartbeat.

Magnesium-rich foods include whole grains, beans (legumes), sea vegetables, vegetable greens, and especially "super green foods" such as chlorella, barley grass, wheat grass, blue-green algae, and other micro-algae.

BROWN RICE

Brown rice contains an abundance of nutrients, including magnesium, before it is processed into white rice. Unlike the west, many Asian countries only partially mill the rice, leaving many more nutrients intact. Asian medicine recognizes brown rice's stabilizing effect on blood sugar. Many of the nutrients in brown rice are contained in the outer coating, or rice bran, which is lost in milling it into white rice. This coating "has rather remarkable effects on lowering blood sugar levels. In addition to reducing blood-sugar levels, <u>rice bran is thought to be one of the most nutrient dense substances ever studied</u>. It embodies over 70 antioxidants that can protect against cellular damage and preserve youthfulness." [13] Rice bran contains an abundance of B vitamins and trace minerals. Among its abundance of antioxidants are glutathione peroxidase, superoxide dismutase, coenzyme Q_{10}, proanthocyanadins, and gamma-oryzanol. "Alpha lipoic acid, a polyphenol antioxidant, promotes liver restoration, slows the aging process and converts glucose to energy." The rice bran is also rich in lecithin, a phospholipid continually produced by the liver. It is vitally important "for proper function of the brain (making up 30% of the dry weight of the brain), nerves and cell membranes." [14]

A note about grains and legumes: Most grains and legumes contain phytic acid, which is known to bind with minerals, making them unavailable to the body. For this reason, grains such as brown rice should be soaked overnight and the soak water poured off before cooking.

DAIRY PRODUCTS

Milk and milk products have a lot to offer in the way of nutrients. They are rich in the fat-soluble Vitamins A, D, E, and K, the water-soluble Vitamins B and C, as well as minerals and trace minerals. Unfortunately, the milk you get at most supermarkets has lost most of its nutrients in processing, while a lot of junk has been added to it.

Modern farming is geared toward quantity over quality. Today's cows have been genetically bred and fed to produce three to four times the milk compared to cows a century ago. Twenty-first century cows have abnormally active pituitary glands that over-stimulate the production of milk and growth hormones.

The freak pituitary cow is prone to many diseases. She almost always secretes pus into her milk and needs frequent doses of antibiotics. Another serious problem with today's dairy methods is the feeding of high-protein soybean meal to the cows, which stimulates them to produce large quantities of milk but contributes to a high rate of mastitis and other problems that lead to sterility, liver problems, and shortened lives.

So we have sick cows needing antibiotics on an ongoing basis, producing large quantities of low quality milk. How can sick cows produce high quality milk? It's impossible. First off, we need our cows to be fed natural foods. As authors Fallon and Enig state, "The proper food for cows is green plants, especially the rapidly growing green grasses in the early spring and fall. Milk from properly fed cows will contain the Price Factor and cancer fighting CLA as well as a rich supply of vitamins and minerals." [15] The Price Factor here actually refers to Activator X, discovered by Dr. Price. Activator X is a powerful catalyst, which, like Vitamins A and D, helps the body absorb and utilize minerals. CLA, or conjugated linoleic acid, is found in butter from cows raised on rapidly growing grass. It has strong anticancer properties, encourages the build-up of muscle and prevents weight gain. "CLA disappears when cows are fed even small amounts of grain or processed feed." [16]

PASTEURIZATION

Pasteurization is another big problem with most milk bought in stores. It basically "sterilizes" the milk, destroying most (more than half) of its nutrients. With today's modern milking machine, efficient storage, packaging, and distribution, pasteurization is actually unnecessary for the purposes of sanitation. In fact, Fallon and Egan point out:

> All outbreaks of salmonella from contaminated milk in recent decades—and there have been many—have occurred in pasteurized milk. Raw milk contains lactic acid-producing bacteria that protect against pathogens. Pasteurization destroys these helpful organisms; leaving the finished product devoid of any protective mechanism should undesirable bacteria inadvertently contaminate the supply. [17]

In addition to destroying most of the nutrients, pasteurization destroys the enzymes in milk, putting a tremendous strain on the body's digestive mechanism. For these reasons, raw milk is far superior to regular pasteurized milk, not only in terms of processing, but also in farming. Additionally, remember that fats are not a bad thing. They are required by your body, and eating or drinking (in this case) any animal product with some or all of the fat taken out is actually detrimental. As stated earlier, fat aids in the proper assimilation of minerals and protein, and eating the animal protein without the fat can lead to serious deficiencies in essential fatty acids.

Homogenization is the final insult to milk. In this process, fat particles of cream are strained through tiny pores under great pressure. The resulting fat particles are so small that they stay in suspension rather than rise to the top of the milk. This suspension makes the fat and cholesterol more susceptible to rancidity and oxidation, and some research indicates that homogenized fats may contribute to heart disease. [18]

If you like to drink milk, I would encourage you to give raw milk a try and see the difference yourself. Raw milk will have a richer flavor and will be much richer in nutrients as well. It can be found at local food co-ops and natural foods markets.

FRUITS AND VEGETABLES

In the Standard American Diet (S.A.D.), fruits and vegetables could be considered the forgotten food group. Fast food restaurants are always busy with people getting burgers, fries, pizzas, and other high calorie, low nutrient foods. These foods usually have a token piece of vegetable on them, such as a thin slice of unripe tomato and a shriveled single piece of lettuce on a burger. Occasionally, a pickle or an onion might even appear. Surprisingly, these are often all the vegetables many people get in their regular diets. And fruits? Forget it!

Unlike today, our grandparents and great-grandparents' diets consisted almost completely of whole foods with a significant portion being fresh fruits and vegetables. Fruits and vegetables contain an abundance of the different vitamins, minerals, and trace minerals needed to keep us healthy. Additionally, co-factors and phytochemicals increase absorption of other nutrients, protect against disease, and strengthen the immune system.

A diet rich in fruits and vegetables is less taxing on the digestive system, and with its high fiber content, improves elimination as well. As pointed out earlier, green vegetables are also rich in chlorophyll.

Chlorophyll has many important properties and actions such as:

Purification:

- Stops bacterial growth in wounds, and anaerobic yeasts and fungi in the digestive tract.

- Deodorizes: eliminates bad breath and odor.

- Removes drug deposits and counteracts all toxins; de-activates many carcinogens.

Anti-inflammation, which counteracts the following inflammations:

- Sore throat

- Pyorrhea

- Gingivitis

- Stomach inflammation and ulcers

- All skin inflammations

- Arthritis

- Pancreatitis

Renewal:

- Builds blood

- Renews tissue

- Counteracts radiation

- Promotes healthful intestinal flora

- Improves liver function

- Activates enzymes to produce Vitamins E, A, and K [19]

VITAMIN AND MINERAL SUPPLEMENTS

Clearly, the best way to get all of your vitamin and mineral needs met is through a diet rich in whole foods. However, with today's fast-paced lifestyle, eating whole foods regularly is not always possible. If you're one of those people who don't quite have the time to prepare and eat a well-balanced and nutritious diet of mostly whole foods, it's probably a good idea to support your diet with vitamin and mineral supplements. Many good companies are using more whole food sources to provide for your body's vitamin and mineral needs. One supplement I particularly like falls in the super green foods category of micro-algae, which includes spirulina, chlorella, and wild blue green algae. Wheat grass and barley grass also fall in this category of super green foods. Their rich chlorophyll content has many healing and rejuvenating qualities, as mentioned earlier. These micro-algae also have many other powerful immune boosting and body-strengthening qualities.

BASIC DIETARY PRINCIPLES

Dietary health also requires following some basic and time-tested concepts, which are practiced quite extensively especially in Asian and European countries. Asian wisdom says to chew your food thoroughly before swallowing, and to eat only until you are 75-80% full. Here's a funny paradox. Asians are "cursed" with a weaker digestive system genetically than most Americans, so they eat less and are healthier because of it. Americans are "cursed" with a stronger digestive system than Asians, so they eat more and are less healthy because of it. The problem with Americans is that they can get away with overeating without much apparent detriment or distress in the short-term, so they do. But they pay for it later.

Another dietary health concept I have come to appreciate resulted from a trip I made to Italy, and it is demonstrated in most European countries, especially Mediterranean ones. Mealtime is viewed as a time to relax, to linger and enjoy food with family and friends (even in restaurants you are encouraged to take your time). Europeans' meals are joyful occasions filled with laughing, talking, and appreciating their bounty. In the presence of such good humor, digestion works amazingly well, so even with all the pasta, bread, cheese, heavy sauces, and wine, most Europeans remain relatively healthy and maintain a good weight.

Contrast this mealtime with that of the average American, eating on the run, zipping in and out of fast food drive-ins, rushing here, there, and nowhere. No wonder high-blood pressure is epidemic in the United States. The sympathetic nervous system is in overdrive! No wonder depression is epidemic here. Families don't sit around and laugh and talk around meals. People are too busy fulfilling the busy schedules they have created!

FASTING

Fasting is rarely used by the average person. In fact, it's often seen as something only religious or dietary fanatics do. And yet, fasting can often restore a sick person to health faster than almost anything else. When animals become ill or injured, they find a protected place to lie down, rest, and fast. Because digestion requires a tremendous amount of energy expenditure, fasting frees this energy up to be used in healing, cleansing, and revitalizing the body.

Pioneers in health and healing, such as Bernard Jensen, D.C. and Herbert Shelton, M.D., have helped thousands of people get well from many advanced degenerative diseases through supervised long fasts, and they have helped others to become healthier through the use of shorter periodic fasting.

I am not a proponent of long fasts for the average person since prolonged fasting can weaken the body. I prefer moderation in fasting and feasting. Actually feasting has a connotation to overeating, so let's just say fasting and eating. Ideally, we should eat moderately most or all of the time, and skip a meal whenever not really hungry. The best meal to skip is supper because our digestive energies are at their highest around mid-day. If lunch and/or breakfast are skipped, supper should be on the light side. Going to bed on a mostly empty stomach allows the body to heal, cleanse, and rejuvenate during sleep.

Periodic one to three day fasts can cleanse and rejuvenate the body more than most people realize. Fasts are especially a good idea after the holidays or after overeating to give your digestive system a rest and to build up vital energy. If you've never fasted before, try a one-day fast and see how wonderful you feel the next day. This is *not*, of course, recommended for diabetics or people with blood sugar problems.

Plenty of good, clean water should be taken during any fast. I do not recommend "juice fasts" because they can really cause blood sugar levels to swing. The way you come off a fast is perhaps the most important part of fasting. People have died after fasting for a week and then breaking their fast with meat, which throws the body into shock, forcing it to go from a state of rest and rejuvenation into a full sprint. Even with a one day fast, it is wise to break your fast with fruits or vegetables.

SALT

A lot of controversy has surrounded salt for quite a while, but its virtues and value are becoming more commonly known and accepted. First off, I want to make a distinction between common table salt (processed and iodized) and sea salt (the whole food form). In his book *Healing with Whole Foods*, Paul Pitchford tells us that the salt controversy raging for the last 50 years has shown salt to be a true culprit. "However, the salt being tested is not the whole salt used for millennia by traditional peoples but the highly refined chemical variety that is 99.5% or more sodium chloride, with additions of anti-caking chemicals, potassium iodide, and sugar (dextrose) to stabilize the iodine." [20] Sea salt, on the other hand, "contains only about 82% sodium chloride; it contains about 14% macro-minerals, particularly magnesium, and nearly 80 trace minerals." [21]

Contrary to the "prevailing wisdom" of many who advocate a low- or no-salt diet, "Most current guidelines for daily salt consumption recommend about 3,000 milligrams, while the average American takes in 17,000 milligrams, or about $3^1/_2$ teaspoonfuls of highly refined salt each day." [22]

This high intake results from a lot of salt being hidden in (added to) the abundance of processed foods most Americans consume. So not only are most Americans consuming more than five times the recommended daily allowance of salt, but they are also getting the wrong kind—the processed kind. It's no wonder some studies have implicated salt as a culprit in creating ill health!

To understand salt's role in the body, we need to understand the importance of osmotic balance in the body's two "oceans." Our cells have both an ocean of fluid inside them and another ocean of fluid outside of them. Osmotic balance means that the water flow between these two oceans is dependent on the ratio of solutes (solids such as potassium, sodium, and sugar) to solvent (water). An increase in the ratio of solutes inside of the cells will pull water into the cell. This process is called osmosis. The solute that "holds" water in the cells is potassium. Sodium is the primary solute that "holds" (keeps) water outside of the cells, although the body also uses sugar and occasionally even uric acid to keep proper osmotic balance. This osmotic balance is extremely important to ensure that all the body's cells get their fair share of water. Water is responsible for transporting nutrients into the cells and taking waste products out of them. As water passes through the cell membrane, it also generates hydroelectric energy, now thought by Dr. Batmanghelidj and other medical professionals to be the body's primary source of energy.

Proper osmotic balance serves many important purposes. It ensures that all cells receive the nutrients they need (including water, the most important of all nutrients after oxygen) and allows for the efficient removal of waste products, all while generating a tremendous amount of hydroelectric energy. What an amazingly efficient system!

To ensure that all these vital functions can occur, the body regulates blood pressure. If a potassium deficiency occurs, the cells are unable to hold sufficient water and become dehydrated. Potassium is found abundantly in fruits and vegetables; its presence allows fruit to hold on to its water. If there is a sodium deficiency, the body will not be able to "hold" onto its water in the extracellular environment, and water will be released from the body through the urine, also causing dehydration. When the body becomes dehydrated from a lack of water and/or salt, "The brain commands an increase in salt and water retention by the kidneys. This directive of the brain is the reason we get edema when we don't drink enough water." [23] Diuretic drugs work by getting rid of sodium from the body, which is quickly followed by water.

Because of its important role in the body's functions, salt is a valuable ingredient in a daily diet. Here are a few more of salt's virtues:

- "Salt is a strong natural antihistamine. It can be used to relieve asthma by putting it on the tongue after drinking a glass or two of water." [24] A full glass of water should always be taken before putting salt on the tongue.

- "Salt is a powerful enzyme activator." [25]

- "Salt is vital for extracting excess acidity from inside the cells, particularly the brain cells. If you don't want Alzheimer's disease, don't go salt-free and don't let your doctor put you on diuretic medications for too long." [26]

- Salt benefits the kidneys by helping it get rid of excess acidity. "Without sufficient salt in the body, the body will become more and more acidic." [27] It's interesting to note that both salt and water work to clear the body of excess acidity.

- "It [salt] strengthens digestion and contributes to the secretion of hydrochloric acid in the stomach." [28]

- "Salt is vital for maintaining muscle tone and strength." [29]

- "Sun-dried sea salt contains traces of marine life that provide organic forms of iodine." [30] Another great source of iodine as well as other minerals is sea vegetables. People suffering with low thyroid function would do well to increase their intake of sea salt and sea vegetables.

- "Salt is essential for preserving the serotonin and melatonin levels in the brain. In a well-hydrated body, tryptophan is spared and gets into the brain tissue, where it is used to manufacture serotonin, melatonin, and tryptamine—essential antidepressant neurotransmitters." [31] Again, salt and water seem to work hand-in-hand. Both dehydration and salt deficiency result in lower levels of brain tryptophan, the essential amino acid from which the major brain neurotransmitters are manufactured.

- "Salt is vital for the generation of hydroelectric energy in all the cells in the body. It is used for local power generation at the sites of energy need by the cells." [32] Once again, salt and water are working in tandem.

- Salt is a natural hypnotic, and is vital for sleep regulation. [33]

- "Osteoporosis is the result of salt and water shortage in the body." [34] Salts give strength to bone tissue by incorporating salt crystals in the bony matrix.

- "Salt is vital for maintaining sexuality and libido." [35] Salt drives energy deeper into the body and downward, which results in increased sexual vitality. I can see you jumping out of your armchair to run to the store.

Sodium and potassium work together similarly to how calcium and magnesium work together. Both pairs have an antagonistic, yet synergistic relationship. In other words, calcium causes muscle contraction while magnesium causes muscle relaxation. And yet, the two work in tandem to maintain normal muscle tone, and magnesium aids in calcium metabolism. Similarly, sodium (salt) and potassium work to keep an osmotic balance—one keeps water inside the cells and the other keeps it outside of the cells. As salt has the quality of driving energy downward in the body and "grounding" a person, potassium promotes upward and outwardly expanding energy. Salt strengthens a person physically and mentally/emotionally, giving him or her self-confidence, a positive self-image and security. But in excess, it can cause kidney damage, fear, and rigidity in the pelvis and the legs. Ultimately, both sodium and potassium are necessary for the proper balance physically and spiritually (mentally/emotionally).

As stated earlier, the general daily amount recommended is 3,000 milligrams—3 grams or half a teaspoon. Individual needs vary based on the amount of water consumed, the temperature outside (more salt and water is required in hotter climates), and a person's level of activity or exercise. Generally, Dr. Batmanghelidj recommends ¼ teaspoon of salt per quart of water consumed. I believe if people consume a diet rich in vegetables, they will fill most of their sodium needs through their diets because many vegetables such as cucumbers and celery are rich in sodium. Rather than taking salt separately (with water), sprinkling it over foods moderately should give the body sufficient salt.

SUGAR AND CAFFEINE

Sugar and caffeine, typically found in sodas and coffee drinks, are among the worst offenders to your body's health, and because of their popularity, it is important to understand why. Dr. Batmanghelidj relates some statistics regarding soda's booming popularity:

> A report published in the magazine *The Nation*, April 27, 1998, stated that the most conservative estimates have children and teens guzzling more than 64 gallons of soda a year, an amount that has tripled for teens since 1978, doubled for the 6-11 set, and increased by a quarter for under-5 tots (from a 1994 survey by the Agriculture Department). The Soft Drink Association surveyed the use of soft drinks in hospitals in America and found 85% served sodas with their patients' meals. [36]

Soft drinks (sodas) and coffee both contain a fair amount of caffeine, but sodas also have a "ton" of sugar. "Cola drinks contain as much as 10% sugar which is 9 times more than the body can metabolize." [37] Both sodas and coffee are consumed abundantly. Many people drink more soda and/or coffee than they do water.

Let's take a look at the individual effects of sugar and caffeine in our bodies. Dr. McBean states, "SUGAR is at last being recognized as a destroyer of health rather than an article of food as was formerly believed. Technically white sugar (C12H220 11) is classified as a drug and not as a food." [38] In other words, it stimulates a chemical response in the body, rather than nourishes. Dr. McBean goes on to say:

> Natural sugar in fruit is in a balanced combination with other constituents that enable it to be assimilated without damage, but when it is separated into the white, crystalline carbon substance called sugar it is converted into alcohol almost immediately after

it is taken into the body and does the same damage that alcohol does. [39]

Again, a vast difference exists between whole foods and processed foods. Whole foods nourish while processed foods have an overall adverse effect in the body.

Sugar dehydrates the cells and leeches the calcium from the nerves, muscles, bones, teeth, and all tissues that are supplied with calcium and other alkaline elements. This loss of calcium occurs because alkaline minerals are required to neutralize the acidity of sugar and eliminate sugar from the body. A serious calcium deficiency is a forerunner of polio. [40]

Perhaps the most damaging ingredient in cola drinks is phosphoric acid. Dr. McBean states, "This acid is a destroyer of the vital calcium supply in the body and even dissolves the enamel on the teeth. Phosphoric acid is made by treating phosphate rock with sulphuric acid." [41]

Calcium is one of the alkaline minerals the body uses to neutralize acidity in the body. It takes 32 glasses of ionized alkaline water to neutralize the acidity of one can of soda. One can imagine the highly acidic condition of many kids who consume several cans of soda a day, and drink very little water.

As for the caffeine in soda, it is an addictive drug because of its direct action on the brain. "Cola is loaded with habit-forming caffeine so that once the victim gets accustomed to the stimulant, he cannot very well get along without it," says Dr. Royal Lee, of the

Lee Foundation for Nutritional Research. "There is only one reason for putting caffeine in a soft drink—to make it habit forming." The same reason naturally applies to coffee. "Caffeine is not only a habit forming drug but it is destructive to the tissues of the stomach, eyes, nerves and kidneys. In fact there is not a part of the body that is not injured by this drug." [42]

Caffeine is a nervous system stimulant. It gives a "pick me up" effect by stimulating the central nervous system to liberate energy from the ATP stores in the brain and body. It also releases energy from calcium in its stored form in the cells. This energy releasing capacity eventually depletes the brain and body of its stored reserves of energy. "It makes the children (and all who drink it) nervous, irritable and high strung and leads to a desire for stronger drink later on." [43]

In nature, the caffeine in the coffee plant protects it from predators by causing stupefaction in the brain, making those animals who consume it more vulnerable to being preyed upon.

Caffeine also has a strong diuretic effect on the kidneys, causing increased urine output, which therefore, makes it a dehydrating agent. In other words, the soda and coffee people often drink in place of water actually leaves them more dehydrated.

ASPARTAME

Aspartame is the sweetening agent used in "diet" sodas and also added to coffee drinks. Like many artificial sweeteners and additives, it has been implicated in causing cancer. "Aspartame is 180 times as sweet as sugar, without any calorie output. It is now in common use because the Federal Drug Administration deemed it safe to use in place of sugar." [44] Upon entering the intestinal tract, it is converted into two neurotransmitter amino acids—aspartate and phenylalanine—and methyl alcohol/formaldehyde. Aspartate and phenylalanine are called neurotransmitters because they have a direct "stimulating effect on the brain, the liver, the kidneys, the pancreas, the endocrine glands, and so on." [45] Dr. Batmanghelidj feels that aspartame, due to its stimulatory effect on the reproductive organs and breasts "may well be implicated in the rise in the rate of breast cancer in women." [46]

ALCOHOL

Alcoholic beverages are consumed throughout the world by most cultures and societies, with many people in these cultures living long and healthy lives. Red wine is even said to promote heart health, through its anti-oxidant qualities found in the molecule resveratrol. Like anything, moderation is essential to good health. Those who drink 1 to 2 glasses of wine a day are found to live longer and healthier lives than those who drink excessively (no surprise), but interestingly, they also live longer than those who do not drink at all.

There are, however, some things to be aware of, in regards to alcohol's effects in the body:

Alcohol causes brain-cell dehydration, by inhibiting the action of vasopressin. (We discussed earlier how vasopressin acts like a showerhead to push water into the cells.) This is the main cause of hangovers, and can often be prevented or mitigated by drinking sufficient water.

- Alcohol is known to cause a deficiency of the B vitamins, trace minerals and the amino acid glutamine.

- Alcohol causes dehydration, by forcing the kidneys to flush water out of the body.

- Alcohol produces free radicals.

- Alcohol is a depressant and should not be consumed by those who are already depressed.

- Alcohol can cause liver damage, impotence, and suppress the immune system.

- Through dehydration, alcohol promotes the secretion of the body's natural endorphins. This may be the factor that causes alcohol addiction.

- Alcohol causes an across-the-board inhibition of all brain functions, with the brain's inhibitory centers being depressed first.

In this information-packed chapter, I have focused on what I consider the most important facts necessary for you to make knowledgeable decisions about your diet and nutrition; you should now have a firm understanding about which specific nutrients are vital for your health and which substances are detrimental to your body's well-being. The bottom line is that whole foods are rich in nutrients while processed foods are nutrient-poor and loaded with toxins and adverse substances. Additionally, nutrients in whole foods work together, enhancing absorption, assimilation, and even their functioning in the body. Whole foods are even better when they are organic. Organic foods are simply those foods raised without the use of inorganic fertilizers, antibiotics, pesticides, and other harmful chemicals. These foods are raised with more care and concern for the environment and animals (for meat or dairy products), leading to greater sustainability in the long-term, as well as a more nutrient-rich food in the present. Organic food sections are growing, even in big chain supermarkets, as consumers become better informed and more aware of whole and nutrient-rich foods' health benefits.

In the next chapter, we'll look at another major factor for good health—chiropractic.

CHAPTER NINE

CHIROPRACTIC

Healing comes from above down, and inside out.
— **B.J. Palmer, D.C.**

Chiropractic is probably the most misunderstood, under-utilized, and yet most powerful healing art in existence. Statistics say that less than 10% of the population goes to a chiropractor. Although chiropractic is becoming more widely accepted, it's amazing to me that so few people see a chiropractor on a regular basis. Years ago, a chiropractic colleague posed the question, "If someone told you that you could never receive another chiropractic adjustment for the rest of your life, how would you feel?" My immediate thought was that I would be devastated! Let me tell you my story.

I was fortunate to grow up in Hawaii, on the beautiful island of Kauai. However, when I was quite young, I had several injuries to my neck and back. When I was about five years old, my mother and I were in a car accident where our car was hit from behind pretty hard; my forehead slammed into the dashboard—they were a lot more solid back then (hard metal with no cushion). A few years later, a playmate of mine was holding me upside down by the ankles and lost his grip. I landed square on my head. OUCH!! To top it off, when I was in the third grade, I took swimming lessons. One of the "rules" was that if a person could swim a certain distance—I forget how far it was, maybe a mile—he or she was allowed to dive off the high board. (Looking back, that is such a ridiculous criterion for that privilege). Anyway, I climbed up the ladder and walked the plank (diving board) with no instruction at all. When I dove (head first, of course) and entered the water, my head was turned to one side (rotated), and I felt and heard a big crack, along with seeing stars. It's a wonder I didn't pass out and sink to the bottom. I swam, or rather struggled, to the side of the pool and hung on in a stupor.

Around the eighth grade, I remember waking up one night with severe, sharp neck pain, and whenever I turned my head to the left, I could barely turn it more than 10 degrees before a sharp pain would radiate into my left arm. This pain became increasingly more frequent until I was afraid I would have to suffer a lot of severe, crippling pain for the rest of my life! What was I going to do? What could I do? I was in a panic.

When I finally told my mom about the pain, she took me to the medical doctor. He suggested I wear a rigid neck support for about nine months. I was about 13 or 14 years old at the time, playing

Little League like most kids my age. Obviously, I couldn't play baseball while wearing a cervical collar. I asked him what a cervical collar would do for me, and whether my neck pain would be gone after nine months. He replied that the collar would stabilize my neck and reduce the inflammation, but he could not guarantee that this great inconvenience would get rid of my neck pain. My intuition as a kid was pretty good. I couldn't see myself wearing a collar for nine months, during which time I would have no life as a kid at all. And I saw no point in it when the doctor gave me little promise of becoming free of neck pain. So I decided against it.

Back in the 1970s (I'm dating myself, but for a worthy cause), it was common to see people who had been involved in a minor fender bender wearing a cervical collar. Today, you almost never see a person wearing a cervical collar unless he has fractured a neck bone. Why is this? Because it is now common knowledge (even among the medical profession) that immobilizing a joint is the worst thing you can do for it (unless it is unstable from a fracture). Rather than reducing inflammation and muscle spasm as the doctor suggested at the time, the opposite would occur…more inflammation and muscle spasm! Chalk one up to my kid's intuition!

Finally, my mom told me about a chiropractor her friend was seeing for her back pain. I said, "What's a chiropractor?" She said she really didn't know, but her friend had said the chiropractor had helped her. Since I was pretty desperate, I said I would try anything! Within two months of seeing the chiropractor regularly, I felt relief.

I was thrilled! I had my life back! This wonderful chiropractor talked to me about chiropractic philosophy, and he encouraged me to go to chiropractic school. I thought about how fulfilling it would be to help other people like myself who were suffering needlessly, so I soon decided on my new career path. I would be a doctor of chiropractic!

Chiropractic has a rather interesting history. In 1895, a physician named D.D. Palmer had a janitor who was 90% deaf. This janitor, Harvey Lillard, could only hear loud sounds vaguely. When asked, Mr. Lillard agreed to let Dr. Palmer examine him. Dr. Palmer palpated (felt) an irregularity in Harvey's spine and asked permission to try and correct it manually, to which Mr. Lillard agreed. The story goes that after his "adjustment," Mr. Lillard got up from the table and could suddenly hear the sounds coming from the street. His hearing was fully restored after three adjustments to the upper thoracic spine. This first adjustment was the beginning of chiropractic, which would go through a long and difficult birth process.

Dr. D.D. Palmer quickly realized the amazing healing power of a chiropractic adjustment ("chiro" meaning "hands" in Latin, and "practic" meaning "to apply"). Eventually, he started the first chiropractic school, the Palmer College of Chiropractic in 1897 in Davenport, Iowa. Once his son, B.J. Palmer, a sort of genius who had the idea for the partitioned cafeteria trays and patented it, helped to develop chiropractic, its popularity began to grow; more and more people attended the chiropractic school, and the public started flocking to chiropractors as "miraculous" healings took place. This popularity soon gained the medical profession's attention, but rather than be open-minded or scientific enough to observe chiropractors' results, it condemned chiropractors and enlisted the "authorities" to put chiropractors in jail. To this day, chiropractic and its practitioners continue to be slandered by the medical profession.

Not until 1987, when Chester Wilk, D.C. and five co-plaintiffs filed the Wilk's et al anti-trust suit against the AMA (American Medical Association) and won, did chiropractic become more widely accepted and respected as a healing profession. However, chiropractors are still viewed by the public as a whole to be less credible than medical doctors. How many chiropractors have heard their patients innocently say, "I'm going to see my 'real' doctor tomorrow"? Initially, this viewpoint puzzled me. M.D. stands for medical doctor. D.D.S. stands for doctor of dentistry, and D.C. stands for doctor of chiropractic. And yet, how many chiropractors have been called Mr. or Mrs. after people learn they are chiropractic physicians? A medical doctor or even a dentist would never be addressed as Mr. or Mrs. It's not that I'm whining here. I'm just pointing out an underlying bias that the public holds toward chiropractors and chiropractic.

Where did this bias come from? It comes from the media, which is controlled by moneyed interests, such as the pharmaceutical industry and the AMA. As Jerry Mander states in *Four Arguments for the Elimination of Television*, "Only the largest corporations in the world have access to network television time because it can cost $120,000 per minute while reaching 30 million people." [1]

The media controls what people see and hear. Media experts know that our brain learns in one of two ways. It learns either through association or repetition. If you see and hear something enough, you will subconsciously accept it as a truth. Look at the sitcom "Two and a Half Men." It might be funny, but it totally depreciates a chiropractor's credibility. While people are laughing, their subconscious mind is associating chiropractors with a struggling nerd in a joke of a profession. By the way, ever wonder why it's called a TV "program"? Because *you are being programmed!* Needless to say, I no longer watch television. Besides, it has adverse health effects. Don't take my word for it—read Jerry Mander's *Four Arguments for the Elimination of Television.*

Between all the misunderstanding and the programmed subconscious bias toward chiropractic, it's no wonder less than 10% of the population uses chiropractic care.

My aim in this chapter is to clear up many of these misconceptions so more people can enjoy the tremendous benefits of regular chiropractic care.

The best place to start is with chiropractic philosophy. One of the principles of chiropractic is that *healing comes from above down, and inside out.* I can hear you thinking, "Why should I care about philosophy?" You should care because philosophy translates into practical application and its end result is your health. For instance, let's look at the diametrically opposed philosophy of the medical profession which says that disease (and health) comes from outside in.

It says or acknowledges nothing about the internal environment that creates the perfect breeding grounds for disease to thrive. Instead, it attempts to fight disease through the use of antibiotics. This approach to treating illness has directly, if not intentionally, resulted in the medical profession and pharmaceutical companies creating "super-bugs," viruses resistant to all medications.

Chiropractors, with their *above down, and inside out* philosophy, recognize that disease can only thrive or survive in an unhealthy environment. In this way, chiropractic is more in alignment with nature, rather than at odds with it.

Now let's take a look at the physiology that supports this view, and delve more deeply into the meaning of *Healing comes from above down, and inside out*. This saying has both a physical and a metaphysical meaning. The metaphysical meaning implies a higher intelligence, which chiropractors call "Innate Intelligence." Innate Intelligence coordinates and controls the healthy functioning of the body through the physical organs of the brain and nervous system. Pause and think for a moment about all the innumerable chemical reactions going on in your body every second. Who's behind the controls? It certainly isn't you, the personality, thank God. Obviously, some great or divine intelligence is maintaining your body in a state of optimal health.

So why do we get sick if there's some divine intelligence running the body? The answer is, just as health comes from above down and inside out, so does disease. Chiropractic philosophy says that much of disease is due to interference in communication between the cells of your body and Innate Intelligence; more specifically, nerve interference. I'll get into the "subluxation above atlas" (your stinking thinking) more in depth in the Mind-Body-Connection chapter, which is the other way Innate Intelligence is prevented from maintaining your body's state of health.

But for now, let's focus on nerve interference. People think of chiropractors as back doctors. But in actuality, we make spinal corrections to remove nerve interference. So in essence, you could say we are more like neurologists, or spinal neurologists. Many of you may have heard the term "subluxation." It's a chiropractic term that simply means nerve interference produced by joint dysfunction. Joint dysfunction occurs when a joint has lost its full and free range of motion.

So what causes the joint dysfunction that produces nerve interference? In a word, stress. Remember, there are three sources of stress: physical, mental/emotional, or chemical. To demonstrate, let's talk about how physical stress produces nerve interference. Physical stress can be due to acute trauma, or chronic strain. When one of these occurs, the body alerts the brain through the warning signal of pain. This warning causes muscle spasms in the injured area to protect it from further harm. It is this muscle spasm that "locks up" the joint, or causes joint dysfunction.

Within two weeks (just about the time you're out of pain and say, "I'm all better now"), the joint dysfunction, which remains, starts to cause the joint to degenerate. Initially, muscles and ligaments develop fibrotic scar tissue in the body's attempt to stabilize the aberrant joint motion. This tissue causes even more joint dysfunction (lack of normal mobility), and becomes a vicious cycle of dysfunction and degeneration. In degeneration's later stages, the body lays down calcium, sort of like pouring concrete to stabilize an area. A chiropractor I know calls this degeneration process the body's Plan B. Plan A is the body's warning system of pain, crying out for its leader (you) to correct the problem. The problem isn't the pain. It's the joint dysfunction causing the pain. Chiropractors adjust the spine to correct joint dysfunction and remove nerve interference, thereby relieving the pain and addressing the true cause.

What about the connection between the spine, the nervous system, and your health? Let's get into the spine's physiology (how things function) and pathophysiology (how things break down). Spinal joints have two kinds of receptors: mechanoreceptors and nociceptors. Mechanoreceptors fire when joints move, giving your body sensory information of your position in space. This information is what allows a major league hitter to connect with a 96 mph fastball. Nociceptors fire when joints are immobilized as in a subluxation (when there is joint dysfunction). Mechanoreceptors and nociceptors fire in opposition; when one fires, the other is inhibited. A healthy functioning joint should have only mechanoreceptors firing, except when trauma is experienced.

A subluxation causes nociceptors to fire *pain* signals to the brain. It's sort of like the space-craft radioing in to say, "Houston, we've got a problem." The brain then sends messages back down the spinal cord and through the spinal nerves, causing the body to respond accordingly. These *pain* signals, however, are filtered out as they go up the spinal cord. Imagine what a neurotic mess you'd be if your conscious brain were bombarded by these *pain* signals all the time. Your survival chances would go down dramatically. For this reason, your body, in its infinite wisdom, filters out the *pain* signals, and research shows that we "feel" the pain (consciously) only 10% of the time. The point is that even when you may not be feeling any pain, your body could be sending distress signals to your brain constantly, to which your brain (and consequently your body) responds.

A great example of the body's response to nerve interference occurred in a young boy who was brought to me by his mother. Chiropractic had given her complete relief from headaches that had plagued her for years, so she wondered whether chiropractic could also help her son. Shortly after he turned two, he developed a chalazon on his left eyelid. A chalazon looks like a cross between a boil, a pimple, and a sty. His chalazon was about the size of a pea. A few months after the boy developed the chalazon, his medical doctor said, "We have to cut it out." His mother acquiesced, and they cut it out. But three weeks later, it was back. She complained to the doctor that it had returned, to which he replied, "Yes, that happens sometimes. We could try cutting it out again though." The mother was very upset that her young boy had gone through the trauma of surgery, only to have the chalazon return; she decided there was no way she would let the doctor cut it out again—especially since he couldn't promise it wouldn't just return. When she brought her son to me, I palpated his neck and found a subluxation of the atlas—the top bone in the neck—whose nerves go to the eyes. I adjusted the boy's atlas and told his mother to bring him back the following week for another visit. When they returned three days later, I walked into the room, looked at the boy, then at his mom and said, "It's gone!" She replied, "Yes, it was gone within 24 hours of the adjustment." Even I was amazed. In the five years since, the chalazon has never returned.

What does this mean in practical terms for your health? To answer that, we need to learn a little more anatomy and physiology. Stay with me, because we are almost there.

Your autonomic nervous system is actually divided into two systems, sympathetic and parasympathetic. These systems work in opposition. When one is activated or stimulated, the other is suppressed or inhibited. The sympathetic nervous system is primarily engaged with physical activity, especially in a fight or flight survival mode. The parasympathetic nervous system is primarily engaged to increase digestion and in the body's healing and reconstruction in times of rest. Generally, the sympathetic nervous system speeds things up. It increases heart rate, respiration, blood sugar levels, blood pressure, and the production of histamine and corticosteroids (stress hormones) while suppressing digestion and the body's ability to heal itself. For this reason, we are advised to wait at least 45 minutes after meals before engaging in strenuous activity. It may also be the reason why allergies and asthma (due to histamine production) often respond so well to chiropractic care. Normally, these two systems work in a state of homeostasis, or balance. When you're more physically active, your sympathetic nervous system predominates. When you're digesting or resting, your parasympathetic nervous system predominates.

In the event of nerve interference from subluxation, your brain responds to the body's distress signals by increasing sympathetic activity, mainly in the area of the subluxation. (Remember that 90% of the time, when you don't feel any pain, your brain is still getting the distress calls, and your brain stem is responding to those signals.) Picture this: It's late at night when you are woken by a sound downstairs. You jump out of bed and strain your ears, listening for the sound of an intruder. Your heart rate, respiration, blood sugar levels, and blood pressure go up, and the stress hormones preparing you for fight or flight are pumping through your body.

Imagine this same process going on continually (to a smaller degree) when you have a subluxation. The distress calls (*pain* signals) continually hitting your brain put your body in a constant state of alarm and stress (increasing sympathetic activity), while shutting down digestion and healing of body tissues (parasympathetic activity). Therefore, as a chiropractor will tell you, a healthy spine is imperative to a healthy body. Certainly, other causes of disease exist, but if a subluxation is present, it is definitely causing less than optimal health in your body.

In conclusion, here is one more analogy. Virtually everyone visits a dentist to care for his or her teeth, and rightfully so, because without your teeth, you couldn't chew your food. But less than ten percent of the population uses a chiropractor. A dentist takes care of the bones in your mouth (teeth), while a chiropractor takes care of the bones in your spine. The big difference is that your oral health does not have a direct impact on your nervous system function but your spine does. Your nervous system's health (and consequently that of your body) is directly related to the health of your spine. As Thomas Edison said, "The doctor of the future…will interest his patients in *the care of the human frame*, in diet and in the cause and prevention of disease."

CHAPTER TEN

EXERCISE AND STRESS

A man's health can be judged by which he takes two at a time—pills or stairs.

— **Joan Welsh**

Our ancestors probably never talked about getting exercise because their lives naturally involved a lot of physical activity. Today, most people have very sedentary jobs, so they need to have exercise in their routines in order to stay healthy. Another difference between our ancestors and us is the kind of stress we have to deal with. In earlier generations, it was mostly the stress of physical survival. In modern society, we have the added stress of processing more information, keeping up with our full calendar of appointments, and being hit with images and artificial light from television, movies, computers, and video games.

Stress, as a whole, activates the sympathetic nervous system.

Generally, it gears you up for physical activity. When more strongly stimulated, it's about survival, and fight or flight. Many people, unaware of it, are functioning constantly in this fight or flight mode. In the last chapter, we talked about the autonomic nervous system, and we got into the differences between sympathetic and parasympathetic activity. Here, we'll get into the chemistry of stress a bit more, so we can better understand the effects of stress on our body. Then we'll look at the virtues of exercise, and how it relieves stress.

During times of increased stress, the body increases its production of the stress hormones. Endorphins are produced to raise the pain threshold and prepare the body to endure hardship and injury until it gets out of danger. My earlier story about the attorney playing "dodge bullet" exemplifies this point beautifully. Women in labor have raised levels of endorphins to cope with the pain of childbirth. For this same reason, teenagers love scary movies and carnival rides, and thrill-seekers risk their lives. It's all just for a chemical hit.

Cortisone is produced to mobilize stored energy and raw materials to deal with a survival situation. Fat stores are broken down into fatty acids to provide energy. Some proteins are broken down into certain amino acids, needed for the production of neurotransmitters, the building of new proteins, and special amino acids to be burned by muscles. This mobilization of energy and resources works well to get a person through a time of hardship or injury, but it depletes the body of its resources when stress becomes a more chronic state. This phenomenon produces the damage associated with (especially prolonged) stress.

Another tremendous stress to the nervous system comes from viewing television. Here's an excerpt from Jerry Mander's excellent book *Four Arguments for the Elimination of Television.*

> Images on television are not real. They are not events taking place where the person who views them is sitting. The images are taking place in the television set, which then projects them into the brain of the viewer. Direct response to them would therefore be more than absurd. So whatever stimulation is felt is instantly repressed. While McLuhan may be correct that seeing the images stimulates the impulse to move, the impulse is cut off. The effect is a kind of sensory tease, to put the case generously. The human starts a process, then stops it, then starts it again, then stops it, vibrating back and forth between those two poles of action and repression, all of it without a purpose in real life.

> There is mounting evidence that this back and forth action is a major cause of hyperactivity; fast movement without purpose, as though stimulated by electricity. The physical energy which is created by the images, but not used, is physically stored. Then when the set is off, it comes bursting outward in aimless, random, speedy activity. I have seen it over and over again with children. They are quiet while watching. Then afterwards they become overactive, irritable and frustrated. [1]

Needless to say, I no longer watch television. To learn more about television's adverse health effects, I highly recommend that everyone read Mander's *Four Arguments for the Elimination of Television*.

When mental stress is high, exercise dissipates stress by putting the body into action, thereby providing a release for the pent up stress. It seems that if a person is stressed but inactive, the stress is internalized more. People with office jobs would do well to walk at least half an hour every day before or after work.

Exercise has many health benefits that go beyond the obvious one of a trim and well-muscled physique:

- Exercise increases the production of the body's natural opiates, endorphins, and enkephalins. [2]

- Exercise lowers blood pressure by opening the capillaries in the muscle tissue, thereby lowering the resistance to arterial blood flow.

- Exercise protects against osteoporosis. The body, being incredibly adaptive, will pull calcium out of the bones if there is insufficient stress on them. Exercise provides that stress, thereby keeping calcium in the bones.

- "Exercise stimulates the activity of the 'fat-burning' enzymes." [3]

- East Asian healing arts practitioners consider exercise to increase the "digestive fire," allowing better absorption and assimilation of nutrients. [4]

- "Exercise lowers blood sugar in diabetics and decreases their need for insulin or tablet medications." [5]

- Exercise increases the levels of two essential amino acids, tryptophan and tyrosine, in the brain. Tryptophan is an essential amino acid that is a precursor to the "anti-depressant" neurotransmitters: serotonin, melatonin, tryptamine, and indolamine. Tyrosine is used in the manufacture of adrenaline, noradrenalin, and dopamine. These neurotransmitters prepare the body for physical action—running, fighting, playing sports, or exercising. The way it prepares itself is by "burning" for fuel the "branched-chain" amino acids that compete with tryptophan and tyrosine. [6]

- Exercise causes the leg muscles to act as a "second heart." When the leg muscles contract, they pump the venous blood back to the heart. Since veins have one-way valves, they allow the blood to go "uphill," and back to the heart. [7]

- "Exercise increases the production of all vital hormones, enhancing libido and heightening sexual performance." [8]

Exercise's greatest benefit is its oxygenation of the body. Not only are capillary beds opened by exercise, but the increased respiration rate and deeper breathing furnish the cells with an abundance of oxygen. As we saw in an earlier chapter, disease cannot establish itself in a high oxygen environment. All cells require oxygen, and they function better when well oxygenated.

I'm going to digress here a bit to discuss the fascinating dance between oxygen, carbon dioxide, water, and all living things. Understanding this dance will help you better to comprehend your body's need for sufficient oxygen, as well as water. This dance is called the oxygen cycle. Plants "inhale" CO_2 (carbon dioxide) like we inhale oxygen. The plant combines the CO_2 with water and the photonic energy from sunlight to produce glucose (its energy source) and "exhales" oxygen into the atmosphere. This process is called photosynthesis. Animals and humans breathe in oxygen, which is used by the mitochondria (the energy generating plants within all cells) to generate adenosine triphosphate, or ATP (our body's energy storage batteries). This process is called cellular respiration, or aerobic (requiring oxygen) respiration. This system functions amazingly. A plant's waste product (oxygen) is our most important nutrient, while our waste product (carbon dioxide) is a plant's most important nutrient. Both processes involve water, oxygen, carbon dioxide, and energy production. Nature is truly amazing! Don't you think we should learn to be in harmony with this Divine Intelligence, rather than at odds with it (the medical approach)?

To summarize this last paragraph, oxygen is needed by our body's cells to produce energy for all cellular functions. Exercise increases the flow of this most vital nutrient to every cell of the body.

Clearly, exercise plays a vital role in a healthy lifestyle. Instead of letting our children spend hours in front of the television and playing computer games, both of which I believe contribute to ADD, ADHD, depression, stress, and other behavioral problems, encouraging children to get exercise will make them all around healthier and happier, more well-adjusted, and better able to enjoy life and face its challenges. Now that we have discussed the physiology of stress, we are prepared to compile all the information we have learned by understanding the Mind-Body Connection.

CHAPTER ELEVEN

THE MIND-BODY CONNECTION

The body is the servant of the mind. It obeys the operations of the
mind, whether they be deliberately chosen or automatically
expressed. At the bidding of unlawful thoughts the body sinks rapidly
into disease and decay; at the command of glad
and beautiful thoughts it becomes clothed with youthfulness
and beauty.
— **James Allen,** *As A Man Thinketh*

A book on health wouldn't be complete without writing about the Mind-Body Connection. Ultimately, the state of your mind may very likely be the most important factor in determining your body's health. The Mind-Body Connection has been the rage in recent years. People like Andrew Weil and Deepak Chopra have written and spoken at length about it, and yet, few people really understand it and its dominant effect upon their health.

This chapter is by no means a "how to" on mastering your mind to improve your body's health. Its purpose is simply to impress upon the reader the absolute certainty that a person's thoughts and attitudes do manifest in the body in an amazingly accurate way. Individuals will express a different manifestation of their attitudes based on their genetic propensities.

Your body is an amazing organism. It's your vehicle, in which you can interact intimately with your environment. Through the senses, you come to know the world in an intimate and personal way. As James Allen wrote a century ago, "the body is the servant of the mind." The mind's purpose is not only to allow you to know the world, but also to know yourself. In other words, your body unerringly reflects your mind or your thoughts. Louise Hay was the first person in recent years to popularize this idea. She related different attitudes to specific illnesses and diseases in the body. She would say that a critical, judgmental attitude would result in arthritis while thoughts of grief, hatred, and long-standing resentment lead to cancer. Louise Hay has written two wonderful books—*Heal Your Body* and *You Can Heal Your Life*—which address practical ways to change your attitudes, to heal your body and your life. I highly recommend them.

Anatomically and physiologically (structurally and functionally), your nervous system is the communication highway between your brain and your body. Through it, your body "talks" to your brain and your brain "talks" to your body. Think of your brain as Houston Central, and your body as the spaceship. The people at

Houston communicate with the astronauts (as well as monitor their equipment) to make sure everything is running fine. If something goes awry or the spaceship's electronic monitoring is showing any equipment dysfunction, Houston can notify the spaceship crew so it can make corrections and adaptations. Clearly, good communication is essential here.

It's the same with your body...with one major difference. That major difference is that the thoughts you entertain every moment are also being communicated to your body. In his book *The Biology of Belief*, Bruce Lipton describes the process as "signal-response." He explains that each cell in our body continually receives signals from the environment through the senses. The cell then re-designs or morphs itself (adapts) according to those signals. This adaptation is ongoing in our bodies. The brain is monitoring the environment through the senses so it may better adapt itself to the environment, thereby increasing its chances for survival.

Additionally, our thoughts about our sensory perceptions, what we *think* about what we see, hear, smell, touch (feel), and taste are also communicated to every cell of our body. The body's cells are also morphing to this "signal." Look at all the numerous studies, tests, and examples of the placebo effect's power. It's well known that people can be cured of fatal diseases by giving them a placebo they believe will help them. Clearly, their beliefs can work some powerful magic within their bodies. A hypnotized subject can feel extreme cold or heat at the hypnotist's suggestion, while the actual temperature around the person is quite comfortable. People with multiple personalities can have one personality suffering from a devastating illness or disease, and the next moment, another personality expresses itself without any sign of the previous personality's disease. Simply amazing! A study from Russia explains this phenomenon:

> According to the findings of the Russian Scientists [the Russian Branch of the Human Genome Project, headed by renowned Dr. Pjotr Garjajev], the genetic code follows the same rules found in human languages. By modulating certain frequency sound patterns on a laser ray, they are able to influence DNA frequency and genetic information. The most interesting aspect of their discovery is that simple words and phrases can work just as well as laser beams. Man can literally reprogram his genetic blueprint through words—which explains why affirmations and hypnosis can have powerful effects on mind and body. [1]

In *The Hidden Messages in Water*, Dr. Masaru Emoto demonstrates clearly the affect of thoughts on water. "Water exposed to 'Thank you' formed beautiful hexagonal crystals, but water exposed to the word 'Fool' produced crystals similar to the water exposed to heavy-metal music, malformed and fragmented." [2]

If water can shape itself according to thoughts, wouldn't our bodies (which are mostly water) do the same? Additionally our body's cells also have DNA, which is continually being imprinted by our thoughts.

DNA, our genetic blueprint, determines the type and quality of proteins the cell will produce. Our DNA is activated by the thoughts we choose to think, consciously or unconsciously. Every thought we have is being sent through our nervous system to every cell in our body. Each thought has its own specific frequency of vibration, and carries specific information along with it. This frequency-specific electrical current triggers the DNA to unravel (open up) specific parts of its genetic code and copy it onto RNA (ribonucleic acid). RNA is the architect's blueprint, which the cell follows to construct "custom-made" proteins out of amino acids. In this way, your body is built to mirror your thoughts.

Additionally, our thoughts trigger the release of neurotransmitters and peptides in the brain, which are absorbed by the body's cells. As Dr. Joe Dispenza states in his book *Evolve Your Brain*, "The most basic, baseline information we need to remember is this: every time we fire a thought in our brain, we make chemicals, which produce feelings and other reactions in the body." [3] Ramtha (Ramtha's School of Enlightenment™) is a 35,000 year old warrior channeled by a lady named J.Z. Knight (who has appeared on "Larry King Live" and "The Merv Griffin Show"). Ramtha has been tested by scientists from the Stanford Research Institute, and was determined to be a separate and unique being from J.Z. Knight, since all vital signs and EEG readings changed dramatically the moment he took control of the body. The scientists were shocked to see a being operating the body from a deep state of delta (normally a deep state of sleep or unconsciousness) in a fully awake and conscious state. Ramtha puts it this way: "Our body hears everything we say and everything we think." [4] Why would the body be set up to hear every thought? What's the purpose of this eavesdropping? To put it simply, your mind is preparing your body for an experience, morphing itself in a unique way that reflects the mind of its leader—you. As Ramtha has said repeatedly, "Attitude is everything!" [5] Brugh Joy, MD has said, "We are in a school for gods—in slow motion—we learn the consequences of thought." [6]

Dr. Andrew Weil, in his book *Spontaneous Remission*, reminds us that an optimistic attitude heals and prevents disease:

> A study of nearly one thousand older adults followed for nine years concluded that people with high levels of optimism had a 23% lower risk of death from cardiovascular disease and a 55% lower risk of death from all causes compared to their more pessimistic peers. [7]

In his well-researched book *The Genie in Your Genes*, Dawson Church relates a study done by Kaiser Permanente, in collaboration with the Centers for Disease Control, called "Adverse Childhood Experiences (ACE)." This study "conducted detailed social, psychological, and medical examinations of 17,421 people enrolled in Kaiser's health plans over a five-year period. The study showed a strong inverse link between emotional well-being, health, and longevity on the one hand, and early life stress on the other." [8]

Specifically, the study found that a person raised in a dysfunctional family had "five times the chance of being depressed than one raised in a functional family," "was three times as likely to smoke," was "at least thirty times more likely to attempt suicide than those who scored low," and "a man with a high score (dysfunctional family) was 4,600% more likely to use illegal intravenous drugs." Additionally, "Ailments more common in those who grew up in dysfunctional families included obesity, heart disease, lung disease, diabetes, bone fractures, hypertension, and hepatitis." [9]

This study demonstrates not only a strong correlation between ACE and habits or life choices, but also between ACE and a greater prevalence of a variety of chronic degenerative diseases.

I end this book with the Mind-Body Connection because I firmly believe (even know), that the mind is the ultimate determinant of one's level of health and well-being. An unhappy mind translates to an unhappy body. A tranquil, joyful state of mind leads to a harmonious and happy body—as within, so without. Again, this is not empty philosophy; I've seen this principle at work in my own body throughout the years.

As an example, just this year—my fiftieth year of life—circumstances caused me to miss a full day (24 hours) of sleep, with no ill result. I was not one bit tired or cranky in the least, but rather, filled with joy and vital energy all day long. I went to bed around ten, and woke up fully refreshed and energized six hours later. Then about a month later, I went on a trip to Argentina—a long plane flight (15 or 16 hours total travel time). A medical physician and friend suggested I take sleeping pills to overcome jet lag and arrive at my destination rested and refreshed. I agreed to take one Ambien six or seven hours before the plane touched down in South America. Nothing happened! I didn't feel drowsy at all and just thought "Oh well." Consequently I missed another full day and night of sleep—again with no ill effect. And again, six or seven hours of sleep and I was ready to go. Several days later, circumstances again caused me to miss another full day and night of sleep, again with no ill effect. So you may have guessed that on the flight home I didn't even try to sleep; instead, I simply read and listened to music. For as long as I could remember (my whole life), I had never missed a full day of sleep without becoming incredibly cranky and tired. In a space of ten days, I had just gone three full days without sleep and felt terrific! Even I was amazed! I am now absolutely convinced that mind is king, and the body dutifully follows and reflects the mind of its leader.

What does this information mean? It means our bodies are continually remolding themselves according to the thoughts we entertain every moment of the day. What's difficult to accept here is the self-responsibility implicated by such an understanding. To accept such a concept implies that we are ultimately responsible for our body's health based upon the thoughts we choose. If this premise is too much of a stretch for you, simply apply the physical principles taught in this book and your health will certainly improve. For those who would like to learn more about the way our thoughts affect our body and much more, there is no greater

place to learn than Ramtha's School of Enlightenment™ (www.ramtha.
com). As a long-time student of the school, I'm still amazed by the way
my body continually molds itself to my current state of mind. Another
great book (a classic actually) written on this topic a full century ago is
As a Man Thinketh by James Allen. A more scientific approach regarding
the physiology of thought into matter is given by Dr. Joe Dispenza in
his highly informative book, *Evolve Your Brain.* Dawson Church's *The
Genie in your Genes* is another excellent book, which will thoroughly
convince you that your thoughts do matter to your body.

CHAPTER TWELVE

YOUR HEALTH REVOLUTION

You say you want a revolution, well you know, we all want to change the world.

— **The Beatles**

Changing the world may be a pipe dream, but revolutionizing your own health is totally doable. You're now armed with the knowledge to take responsibility for your own health. Remember the man I told you about in the introduction to Part One? Being able to "think on his feet" saved his eye; along with the investment he made in a water ionizing machine. It all comes down to applying the knowledge you learned. Recall also that the medical approach to this man's condition would have done absolutely nothing to save his eye. The medical profession is usually excellent at emergency care, but woefully inept at curing diseases, and promoting health.

At this point, I want to address some attitudes surrounding health that I've observed as a physician of 24 years. Young people (through their twenties and even their thirties) don't have to work very hard to feel fantastic, most of the time. They are filled with vital energy, and outside of an occasional flu or cold, appear to be unrestricted (by their body) in their enjoyment of life. They feel invincible! Things change when people hit forty or so. Their poor attitudes and lifestyle habits start to catch up with them. They bemoan their "old age", and long for their youth. All of a sudden, they don't take their health for granted anymore. For those who fall into this category, I want to tell you that it's never too late to turn your health around. My mom enjoys excellent health and vitality at the ripe age of eighty-eight, thanks to a joyful and caring attitude, as well as a wholesome diet. For those who are younger, I encourage you not to take your health for granted, and to start to improve your attitudes and lifestyle habits now, so you can have many more years of unrestricted enjoyment out of life.

One attitude I'd like to address concerns pain. Pain is NOT your enemy; it's your body crying out for you to change something (such as drink more water). Pain is your body's cry for help. It's not there to annoy you, or make you miserable. It's your body's way of letting you know you're making IT miserable. So stop being upset at your body for hurting, and start listening to it. You're the one who is causing it to hurt by your poor lifestyle habits and/or your sour attitudes. Taking responsibility for your health means being real (honest with yourself), looking at what you need to change, and doing it (changing).

Another attitude surrounding pain is the macho attitude of

"ignoring it," or tolerating it because "you're tough." No, you're just (being) stupid. Tolerating pain is NOT a virtue; it's ignorance. Your poor body is pleading with you to change something! Okay…I'll try to scale my passion back a little bit. I think you get the message. The thing is that the medical profession wants you to believe that pain and other symptoms are restricting your enjoyment of life, and so you should take a pill (to suppress the symptoms) so you can continue to enjoy life. That is so ignorant! One of my favorite statements (that I made up) is "Ignorance is bliss…for a little while. And then reality kicks you in the teeth." The reason the medical belief (more like propaganda or dogma) is ignorant is because pain medication allows you to go on continuing to abuse your poor body. It's not the pain that's restricting your enjoyment of life; it's your poor lifestyle habits and attitudes that are catching up with you—and consequently, restricting your enjoyment of life. The only time pain medication is justified or worthwhile (as I see it), is when you've just suffered a traumatic injury (I'm actually very thankful for anesthetics in this instance), or you are in intractable pain from disease. ALL other medications do more harm than good. Over the years, I've noticed that the more medications people are on, the sicker they are. With the knowledge you've gained in this book, you hopefully understand why.

Another attitude I'd like to address is in regards to health fanatics, who are always searching for the latest and greatest—the magic bullet that will cure everything—while ignoring basic health principles. They go from one fad to another, never really understanding anything about any of it. Some "health guru" just told them something was a "cure-all." NOTHING is a cure-all, because not all diseases have the same cause. Just as no one thing will cure all diseases, no one thing will give you radiant health either.

My friend was just telling me the other day about a video he saw on You-Tube that claimed hydrogen peroxide therapy could cure any disease by increasing oxygen levels in the body. What my friend didn't know is that hydrogen peroxide is a powerful free radical (or oxidizing agent), which requires certain catalysts in order for it to decompose into water and oxygen. (If there's anything you want to understand better, Wikipedia is an excellent resource.) By the time hydrogen peroxide has decomposed into water and oxygen, a lot of damage has probably been done through its oxidizing qualities (as a potent free radical). Furthermore, how much of it actually will be decomposed is totally unknown. I'd say many safer ways exist to increase the body's oxygen levels such as regular exercise, breathing more deeply throughout the day, and drinking ionized water. The abundance of hydroxyl ions (-OH) in ionized water readily provides an abundance of free oxygen, with absolutely NO side effects. By the way, hydroxyl ions (-OH) are exactly half of a hydrogen peroxide (H_2O_2) molecule; therefore, they're just a step away from turning into oxygen—no catalyst needed.

The moral of this story is: Stop chasing around for the magic cure. The only "magic cure" for dehydration is to drink more water, and drink less dehydrating agents such as coffee, soda, and alcohol. If you're dehydrated (deficient in the vital nutrient called water), no number of other supplements at a health food store is going to cure your ills. The only "magic cure" for obesity is to eat less and exercise more. Stop complicating things, and get real. Health is not a complicated thing. You just have to be willing to change and let go of your poor lifestyle habits. If you're not willing to stop drinking ten sodas a day, there's no way you're going to be healthy! A good friend I shared my manuscript with took my book to heart and stopped drinking soda (he was only drinking one soda a day) and started drinking more water. After two weeks, he called to thank me for how much better he felt.

Stop believing in things other people say. ("Health gurus" capitalize on gullible people looking for a cure-all.) Stop believing and start knowing, by learning and understanding how your body works, and what it requires to be healthy. Stop acting confused, and start becoming knowledgeable. In this book, I've clearly outlined your body's basic requirements for it to be healthy. If you just apply the simple knowledge contained here, I promise your health will improve significantly.

Another complaint I hear often is that there's so much conflicting information out there, that it's hard to know who or what to believe. *Again, I'm not asking you to believe anything I say;* ***I want you to understand everything*** *I say.* That's why I've discussed physiology and a bit of biochemistry. A health book will do you no good if you don't come away from it with a better understanding of how to improve your health. When you truly understand how your body works, what it requires to be healthy (and why), you'll see through all the lies, propaganda, and misinformation; and you won't be confused anymore.

Okay, so with all the knowledge you've gained in this book, how do you apply it? First, drink more water and less coffee, tea, juice, or soda. Even better, drink ionized water. Just from this change alone, your health will improve tremendously. If you are seriously interested in purchasing a good water ionizer, I believe the Kangen Water™ machines made by Enagic to be the best. They're not cheap, but you certainly get more than your money's worth. They come with a five year warranty, and a life expectancy of fifteen to twenty years. They are listed under the bibliography and resources section at the end of the book. In regards to diet, the more whole foods and the less processed foods you eat, the better your health will be. Shop more at natural foods markets and local co-ops, where most or all of the food is organic. It may cost a little more, but your health will be much better for it. Better still, grow your own food. Stay away from prescription drugs, and you will be so much healthier. Find a great chiropractor, and make that a part of your wellness lifestyle. In my mind, chiropractic is the greatest healing art around. Stay away from vaccines like you avoid the plague, because they are a plague. Get regular exercise, and try to make it something you enjoy doing; that way, you're more likely to stick with it. Get rid of your antagonistic and resentful attitudes because they are sucking the life right out of your body. Cleanse your mind of ill and bitter thoughts, and your body will sing with joy and youthfulness.

I strongly encourage you to keep learning. In the bibliography, you'll find some of the best books and resources to learn more and live a much healthier and happier life.

Congratulations and Bon Voyage!

NOTES

Introduction

[1] Sally Fallon & Mary G. Enig, Nourishing Traditions (Washington D.C.: New Trends Publishing, 2001), p. 5.

PART ONE: Getting Beyond the Programming of Big Medicine

Chapter 1. Healthcare vs. Sickness Care

[1] http://en.wikipedia.org/wiki/Health_care_reform_in_the_United_States

[2] Eleanor McBean, The Poisoned Needle—Suppressed Facts About Vaccination (out-of-print book published as a public service, no publisher or date of publication provided), p. 2.

[3] http://robertreich.blogspot.com/2009/11/harry-reid-and-what-happened-to-public.html

[4] http://www.dailyfinance.com/story/limited-drug-competition-a-prescription-for-extreme-price-increa/19313499/?icid=main|htmlws-main-n|dl3|link3|http%3A%2F%2Fwww.dailyfinance.

com%2Fstory%2Flimited-drug-competition-a-prescription-for-extreme-price-increa%2F19313499%2F

[5] http://www.naturalnews.com/027582_Merck_Vioxx.html

[6] Journal of the American Medical Association April 16, 2008; Vol. 299 No. 15, pp. 1833-1835

[7] The Poisoned Needle, p. 102.

[8] Ibid.

[9] Ibid.

[10] Ibid., p. 104.

[11] Ibid., p. 105.

[12] Ibid., p. 3.

[13] Ibid.

Chapter 2. Your Body (of H2O) and Water

[1] Mu Shik Jhon, The Water Puzzle and the Hexagonal Key, (United States of America: Uplifting Press, 2004), p. 2.

[2] Ibid, p. 39

[3] Ibid., p. 70.

[4] Ibid, p. 71.

[5] Ibid, p. 72.

[6] Masaru Emoto, The Hidden Messages in Water (Hillsboro, OR: Beyond Words Publishing, 2004), xix.

[7] Ibid, xxiii.

Chapter 3. Causes of Most Diseases

[1] Fereydoon Batmanghelidj, Your Body's Many Cries for Water

(USA: Global Health Solutions, Inc., 2008), p. 4.

[2] F. Batmanghelidj, Water for Health, for Healing, for Life (New York: Hachette Book Group USA, 2003), p. 27.

[3] Ibid , p. 20.

[4] Ibid.

[5] Ibid., pp. 23-24.

[6] Ibid, p. 23.

[7] Ibid.

[8] F. Batmanghelidj, Water Cures: Drugs Kill (Vienna, VA: Global Health Solutions, 2003), p. 7.

[9] Mu Shik Jhon, The Water Puzzle and the Hexagonal Key, (United States of America: Uplifting Press, 2004), p. 74.

[10] Cries for Water, p. 39.

[11] Ibid.

[12] Ibid., p. 128.

[13] http://en.wikipedia.org/wiki/Allergy

[14] Your Body's Many Cries for Water, p. 39.

[15] Nourishing Traditions, p. 35.

Chapter 4. The Remedy

[1] Dave Carpenter, Change Your Water, Change Your Life (Bend, OR: Alliance Press, 2009), p. 19.

[2] Mu Shik Jhon, The Water Puzzle and the Hexagonal Key, (United States of America: Uplifting Press, 2004), pp. 60-61.

[3] Ibid., p. 91.

Chapter 5. Heart Disease

[1] Peter Libby, "Atherosclerosis: The New View," Scientific American, May, 2002/November 10, 2008, www.scientificamerican.com/article.cfm?id=atherosclerosis-the-new-view.

[2] Ibid.

[3] Sally Fallon & Mary G. Enig, Nourishing Traditions (Washington D.C.: New Trends Publishing, 2001), p. 5.

[4] F. Batmanghelidj, Water Cures: Drugs Kill (Vienna, VA: Global Health Solutions, 2003), p. 7.

[5] Nourishing Traditions, p. 11.

[6] Ibid, p.12.

[7] http://en.wikipedia.org/wiki/Cholesterol

[8] Nourishing Traditions, p. 12.

[9] Ibid.

[10] Ibid, p. 10.

[11] Ibid, p. 12.

[12] Ibid, pp. 12-13.

Chapter 6. Diabetes and High Blood Pressure

[1] http://en.wikipedia.org/wiki/Diabetes_mellitus

[2] Ibid.

[3] Ibid.

[4] Fereydoon Batmanghelidj, Your Body's Many Cries for Water (USA: Global Health Solutions, Inc., 2008), p. 63.

Chapter 7. Vaccines

[1] John Drake, Vaccination Horror—An Anthology on Important Works on Vaccination Pseudo-science (Fearlesspublishing.net, 2009), p. 21.

[2] Ibid, p. 20.

[3] Ibid, p. 21.

[4] Ibid.

[5] Ibid, p. 20.

[6] Sherri Tenpenny, Saying No to Vaccines (Cleveland, Ohio: NMA Media Press, 2008), p. 30.

[7] Vaccination Horror, p. 27.

[8] Ibid, p. 22.

[9] Ibid.

[10] Ibid, p. 25.

[11] Saying No to Vaccines, p. 31.

[12] Ibid.

[13] The Poisoned Needle, p. 13.

[14] Ibid, p. 71.

[15] Ibid, p. 21.

[16] Ibid.

[17] Ibid, p. 41.

[18] Saying No to Vaccines, p. 47.

[19] Ibid, p. 48.

[20] Ibid, p. 49.

[21] Ibid.

[22] Ibid, p. 54.

[23] Ibid, pp. 188-189.

[24] Ibid, p. 57.

[25] Ibid, p. 56.

[26] Ibid, p. 59.

[27] Ibid, pp. 28-29.

[28] Ibid.

[29] Ibid, p. 37.

[30] Ibid, p. 23.

[31] Ibid, p. 20.

[32] Ibid, p. 7.

[33] Ibid, p. 41.

PART TWO: A Blueprint for Radiant Health and Wellness

Chapter 8. Diet and Nutrition

[1] Paul Pitchford, Healing with Whole Foods (Berkeley, California, North Atlantic Books, 2002), p. 217.

[2] Nourishing Traditions, p. 28.

[3] Ibid.

[4] Ibid, p. 29.

[5] Ibid, p. 10.

[6] Ibid.

[7] Ibid, pp. 14-15.

[8] Ibid, p. 15.

[9] Healing with Whole Foods, p. 8.

[10] Ibid, pp. 8-9.

[11] Ibid, p. 9.

[12] Ibid, p. 10.

[13] Paul Pitchford, Healing with Whole Foods (Berkeley, California, North Atlantic Books, 2002), p. 13.

[14] Ibid, pp. 13-14.

[15] Nourishing Traditions, pp. 16-17.

[16] Ibid.

[17] Ibid, p. 34.

[18] Ibid, p. 15.

[19] Healing with Whole Foods, p. 228.

[20] Ibid, p. 196.

[21] Nourishing Traditions, pp. 48-49.

[22] Healing with Whole Foods, p. 197.

[23] Your Body's Many Cries for Water, p. 152.

[24] Ibid, p. 154.

[25] Healing with Whole Foods, p. 48.

[26] Your Body's Many Cries for Water, p. 154.

[27] Ibid.

[28] Healing with Whole Foods, p. 196.

[29] Your Body's Many Cries for Water, p. 155.

[30] Nourishing Traditions, p. 48.

[31] Your Body's Many Cries for Water, p. 155.

[32] Ibid, p. 157.

[33] Ibid.

[34] Ibid, p. 158.

[35] Ibid.

[36] Ibid, pp. 106-107.

[37] The Poisoned Needle, p. 135.

[38] Ibid, pp. 134-135.

[39] Ibid.

[40] Ibid.

[41] Ibid.

[42] Ibid.

[43] Ibid.

[44] Your Body's Many Cries for Water, p. 109.

[45] Ibid, p. 111.

[46] Ibid, p. 112.

Chapter 9. Chiropractic

[1] Jerry Mander, Four Arguments for the Elimination of Television, (New York, NY: Harper Collins Publishers, Inc., 1978), p. 143.

Chapter 10. Exercise and Stress

[1] Jerry Mander, Four Arguments for the Elimination of Television, (New York, NY: Harper Collins Publishers, Inc., 1978), p. 167.

[2] Your Body's Many Cries for Water, p. 167.

[3] Ibid, p. 165.

[4] Healing with Whole Foods, p. 15.

[5] Your Body's Many Cries for Water, p. 166.

[6] Ibid, pp. 165-166.

[7] Ibid, pp. 166-167.

[8] Ibid, p. 167.

Chapter 11. The Mind-Body Connection

[1] alternativespirituality.suite101.com/article.cfm/dnachanges

[2] Masaru Emoto, The Hidden Messages in Water (Hillsboro, OR: Beyond Words Publishing, 2004), p. 25.

[3] Joe Dispenza, Evolve Your Brain, (Deerfield Beach, FL: Health Communications, Inc., 2007), p. 302.

[4] Ramtha, Ramtha's School of Enlightenment TM

[5] Ibid.

[6] Dawson Church, The Genie in Your Genes (Santa Rosa, CA: www.energypsychologypress.com, 2009), p. 53.

[7] Ibid, p. 73.

[8] Ibid, p. 60.

[9] Ibid.

BIBLIOGRAPHY
AND RESOURCES

Allen, James. *As A Man Thinketh*, (Scotts Valley, CA: CreateSpace, 2009).

Batmanghelidj, Fereydoon. *Water Cures: Drugs Kill* (Vienna, VA: Global Health Solutions, 2003).

Batmanghelidj, Fereydoon. *Water for Health, for Healing, for Life* (New York: Hachette Book Group USA, 2003).

Batmanghelidj, Fereydoon. *Your Body's Many Cries for Water* (USA: Global Health Solutions, Inc., 2008).

Bragg, Patricia and Paul. *Super Power Breathing for Super Energy*, (Santa Barbara, CA: Health Science)

Carpenter, Dave. *Change Your Water, Change Your Life* (Bend, OR: Alliance Press, 2009).

Church, Dawson. *The Genie in Your Genes* (Santa Rosa, CA: www.energypsychologypress.com, 2009).

Colbin, Annemarie. *The Book of Whole Meals*, (U.S.A.: Ballantine Books, 1983).

Dispenza, Joe. *Evolve Your Brain*, (Deerfield Beach, FL: Health Communications, Inc., 2007).

Emoto, Masaru. *The Hidden Messages in Water* (Hillsboro, OR: Beyond Words Publishing, 2004).

Fallon, Sally and Mary G. Enig. *Nourishing Traditions* (Washington D.C.: New Trends Publishing, 2001).

Jensen, Bernard. *Foods That Heal*, (Avery Trade, 1988).

Jhon, Mu Shik. *The Water Puzzle and the Hexagonal Key*, (U.S.A.: Uplifting Press, 2004).

Knight, J.Z. Ramtha, (Yelm, WA: JZK Publishing, 2004).

Mander, Jerry. *Four Arguments for the Elimination of Television* (New York, NY: Harper Collins Publishers, Inc., 1978).

McBean, Eleanor. *The Poisoned Needle—Suppressed Facts About Vaccination* (out-of-print book published as a public service, no publisher or date of publication provided).

Pitchford, Paul. *Healing with Whole Foods* (Berkeley, CA: North Atlantic Books, 2002).

Robbins, John. *Diet for a New America*, (Walpole, NH: Stillpoint Publishing, 1987).

Tenpenny, Sherri. *Saying No to Vaccines* (Cleveland, OH: NMA Media Press, 2008).

ONLINE RESOURCES:

www.enagic.com – source for Kangen Water™ machines

www.Mercola.com

www.naturalnews.com

www.ramtha.com

www.watercure.com

INDEX

B

D

H

O

P

R

S

T

U

V